T0042069

THE 28-DAY PLAN FOR IBS RELIEF

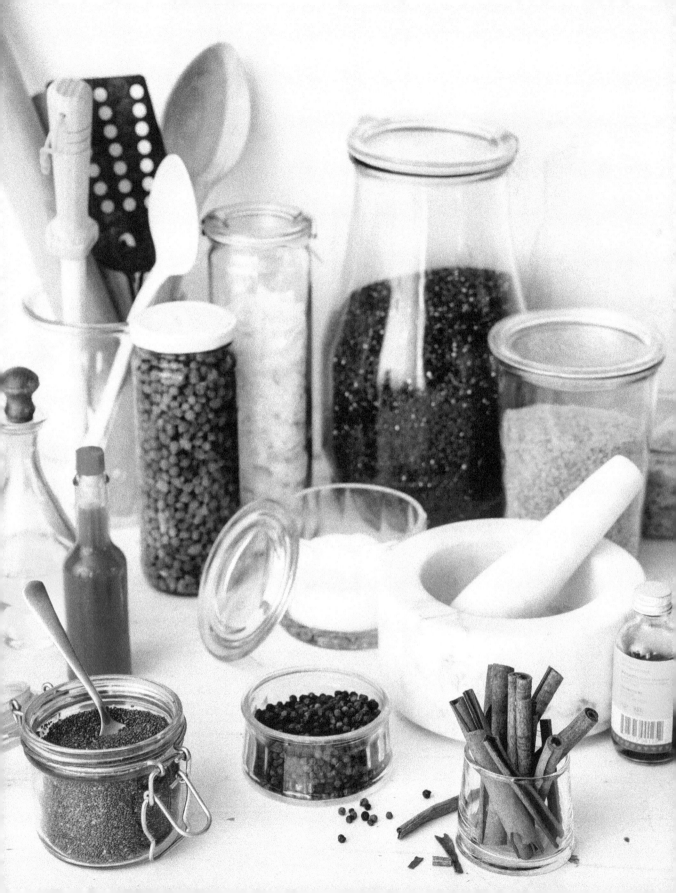

The
28-DAY PLAN
for IBS RELIEF

100 Simple **LOW-FODMAP** Recipes to Soothe Symptoms of **IRRITABLE BOWEL SYNDROME**

Audrey Inouye, BSc, RD and
Lauren Renlund, BASc, MPH, RD

FOREWORD BY JOANNA BAKER, APD

Photography by Annie Martin

ROCKRIDGE PRESS

Copyright © 2020 by Rockridge Press, Emeryville, California

No part of this publication may be reproduced, stored in a retrieval system, or transmitted in any form or by any means, electronic, mechanical, photocopying, recording, scanning, or otherwise, except as permitted under Sections 107 or 108 of the 1976 United States Copyright Act, without the prior written permission of the Publisher. Requests to the Publisher for permission should be addressed to the Permissions Department, Rockridge Press, 6005 Shellmound Street, Suite 175, Emeryville, CA 94608.

Limit of Liability/Disclaimer of Warranty: The Publisher and the author make no representations or warranties with respect to the accuracy or completeness of the contents of this work and specifically disclaim all warranties, including without limitation warranties of fitness for a particular purpose. No warranty may be created or extended by sales or promotional materials. The advice and strategies contained herein may not be suitable for every situation. This work is sold with the understanding that the Publisher is not engaged in rendering medical, legal, or other professional advice or services. If professional assistance is required, the services of a competent professional person should be sought. Neither the Publisher nor the author shall be liable for damages arising herefrom. The fact that an individual, organization, or website is referred to in this work as a citation and/or potential source of further information does not mean that the author or the Publisher endorses the information the individual, organization, or website may provide or recommendations they/it may make. Further, readers should be aware that websites listed in this work may have changed or disappeared between when this work was written and when it is read.

For general information on our other products and services or to obtain technical support, please contact our Customer Care Department within the United States at (866) 744-2665, or outside the United States at (510) 253-0500.

Rockridge Press publishes its books in a variety of electronic and print formats. Some content that appears in print may not be available in electronic books, and vice versa.

TRADEMARKS: Rockridge Press and the Rockridge Press logo are trademarks or registered trademarks of Callisto Media Inc. and/or its affiliates, in the United States and other countries, and may not be used without written permission. All other trademarks are the property of their respective owners. Rockridge Press is not associated with any product or vendor mentioned in this book.

Interior and Cover Designer: Lisa Forde
Art Producer: Michael Hardgrove
Editor: Marjorie DeWitt
Production Editor: Kurt Shulenberger

Photography © 2019 Annie Martin

Food styling by Emily Cooper

Author photo courtesy of © Garrett Rokosh

ISBN: Print 978-1-64152-886-3 |
eBook 978-1-64152-887-0

R0

This book is dedicated to anyone who has suffered from IBS and to the worldwide community of FODMAP specialist dietitians working hard to support them.

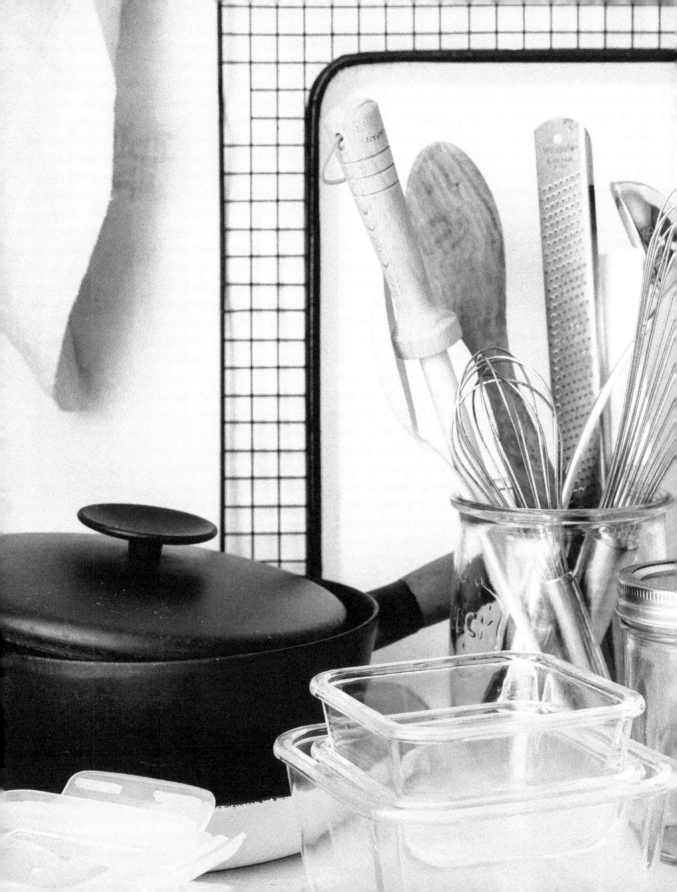

Contents

Foreword

HI, I'M JO, AND I'M A DIETITIAN WHO LOVES FOOD. I'M ALSO SOMEBODY who has suffered with food intolerances and IBS for longer than I can remember. I know what it's like to live with unpredictable (and embarrassing!) gut upsets. Before finding the low-FODMAP diet, I felt like my life was out of control. It was not only affecting my work life; it was also affecting my social life and marriage and preventing me from being the type of mom I wanted to be.

The low-FODMAP diet was a game changer for me. Like three out of four people who have IBS and follow a low-FODMAP diet, I experienced a consistent and significant improvement in my gut. Within about a week, I didn't need to loosen my jeans in the car on the way home, and for almost the first time in my life, I was using the toilet normally. This was the beginning of my FODMAP journey.

Of course, the low-FODMAP diet isn't something that you stay on for life. I moved forward and identified exactly which FODMAPs I tolerate well and which ones I can enjoy occasionally. And then there's garlic, which in my world has its own category of evil. Of course, these results will be different for everyone, but what is consistent is the increased knowledge that the low-FODMAP diet has given me. And, at the end of the day, knowledge is power. It was this experience that motivated me to complete the Monash training for dietitians and step away from my hospital role to focus my career on helping people with IBS learn to love food again.

The low-FODMAP diet is now the most researched and most effective way of managing IBS, but it is a complex process. Not only does it limit lists of seemingly random foods, but also there are four different groups of FODMAPs and further subgroups as well. Getting a list of foods to eat or avoid is really just the beginning. A low-FODMAP diet is much more about thresholds and serving sizes than it is black and white. Many foods are okay in one serving size but at a larger serving size become problematic. Then there is navigating reading labels and ingredient lists and eating out, not to mention the intricacies of how FODMAP levels are affected by food processing. Even for dietitians, this makes the FODMAP diet a specialty area that requires further training to master.

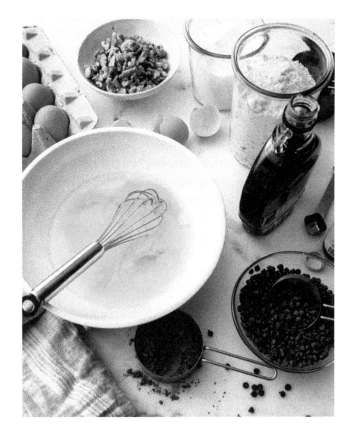

A dietitian who is Monash-trained (the FODMAP diet was first developed by researchers at the University of Monash in Melbourne, Australia) will ensure that you get the low-FODMAP diet right for your needs, will guide you through identifying your triggers, and, crucially, will make sure that what you eat provides the value you need to function on all cylinders every day.

I'm now excited to be part of a wonderful network of FODMAP-trained registered dietitians all over the world. Audrey and Lauren, who wrote this book, continue to inspire me with their compassion, practicality, and down-to-earth approach, not to mention their delicious recipes! I love the idea that food should be simple to prepare and delicious to eat and help you feel good inside and out. Living with food intolerances or IBS shouldn't mean missing out on yummy food, and the recipes in this cookbook fit the bill perfectly. I'm thrilled to be part of this project!

Joanna Baker, MDiet, BHSc, APD, RN, owner of Everyday Nutrition

Introduction

HELLO! WE ARE SO HAPPY YOU DISCOVERED OUR LOW-FODMAP COOKBOOK for IBS. Too many people with IBS have lost their love of food, so we are giving you the best from our kitchens and our hearts so that IBS doesn't hold you back any longer.

We (Lauren and Audrey) are among the first dietitians in North America to specialize in the low-FODMAP diet. Collectively, we have helped thousands of people with IBS and digestive symptoms. We are also good friends. Our friendship started in December 2016 when we both had new private practices specializing in IBS and the low-FODMAP diet. We connected over Facebook and soon realized that only a handful of other dietitians in North America had the same specialty. Living on opposite sides of Canada, we started consulting with each other about complicated patients, ingredient lists, and our new favorite recipes. Now here we are three years later, both living in Edmonton and writing a cookbook together for you.

Lauren struggled with digestive issues for many years but wasn't diagnosed with IBS until 2014, after contracting a bad gut bug. She had just started her master's degree and was struggling to keep up in school because of constant IBS symptoms and anxiety. After months of pain and frustration, she bought a book and started the low-FODMAP diet. It was tough to do alone, but she was able to get her symptoms under control, finish her degree, and fulfill her dream of becoming a dietitian. After graduating in 2016, she started a private practice and food blog. She felt empowered by sharing her story and knowing she could help others in similar situations. Creating her own low-FODMAP recipes helped her fall in love with food again. She currently works in community health.

Audrey's career as a dietitian started in 2001. When she later discovered the low-FODMAP diet in her private practice, she was delighted and intrigued by how quickly her patients felt significantly better. It made her feel like a rock star dietitian! Audrey also knew that IBS was complicated and multifactorial and that simply sharing a list of high-FODMAP foods with her patients would not be enough. She set out to learn as much as she could. She completed several training programs, including the Monash FODMAP course for dietitians, which provided her with comprehensive education on the intricacies of the low-FODMAP diet. IBS is now the exclusive focus for Audrey's practice, IBS Nutrition. She continues to test low-FODMAP recipes on her most discerning critics, her husband and three boys.

The low-FODMAP diet is a medical diet that is recommended as a first line of dietary treatment for IBS. It has been shown to provide relief from bloating, abdominal pain or discomfort, constipation, and diarrhea in up to three out of four people with IBS. It was intelligently designed by researchers at Monash University and is best followed with support from a Monash FODMAP-trained dietitian. You don't have to struggle through the diet alone, like Lauren had to do years ago.

In our book, you will discover 100 of our favorite low-FODMAP recipes and our 28-day low-FODMAP meal plan. Since the low-FODMAP diet is complicated enough, our recipes are simple and fast. Your meal plan for each week includes a shopping list and a summary of things to prep before your week starts. We've worked with our worldwide FODMAP specialist dietitian network to ensure every one of the following recipes is reliably low-FODMAP.

As you navigate this book, we hope you feel our words of encouragement guiding you along. We love cooking for our friends and family and have thoroughly enjoyed curating these recipes for you, too.

With much love,

Lauren and Audrey

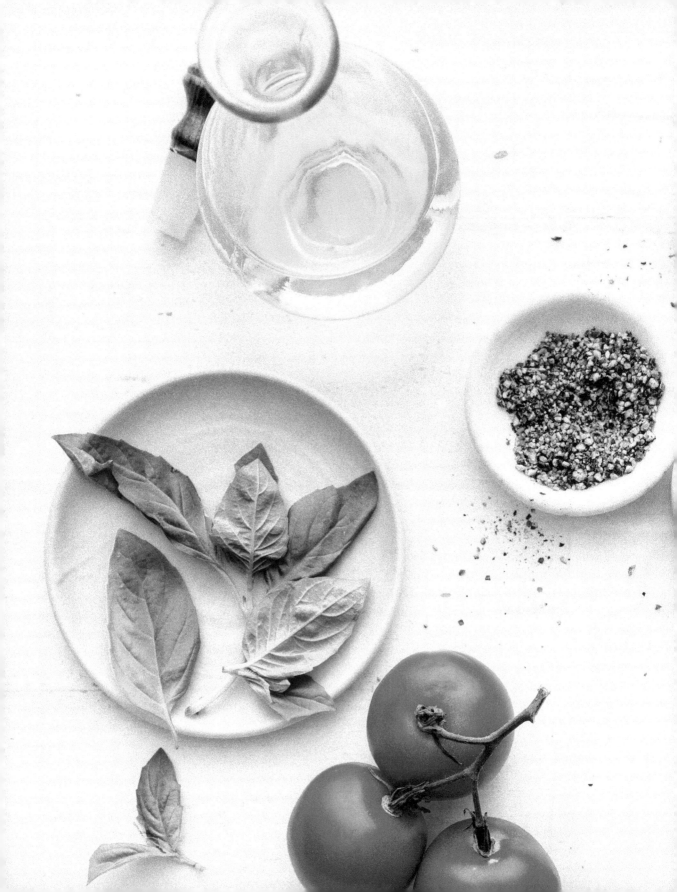

PART ONE

SOLVING FOR IBS

It is easy to feel completely overwhelmed when starting on this journey. An online search may send you in a million different directions and leave you with more questions than answers. That is why we will systematically and succinctly teach you about IBS and how to reduce your food triggers with the most effective diet for IBS, the low-FODMAP diet.

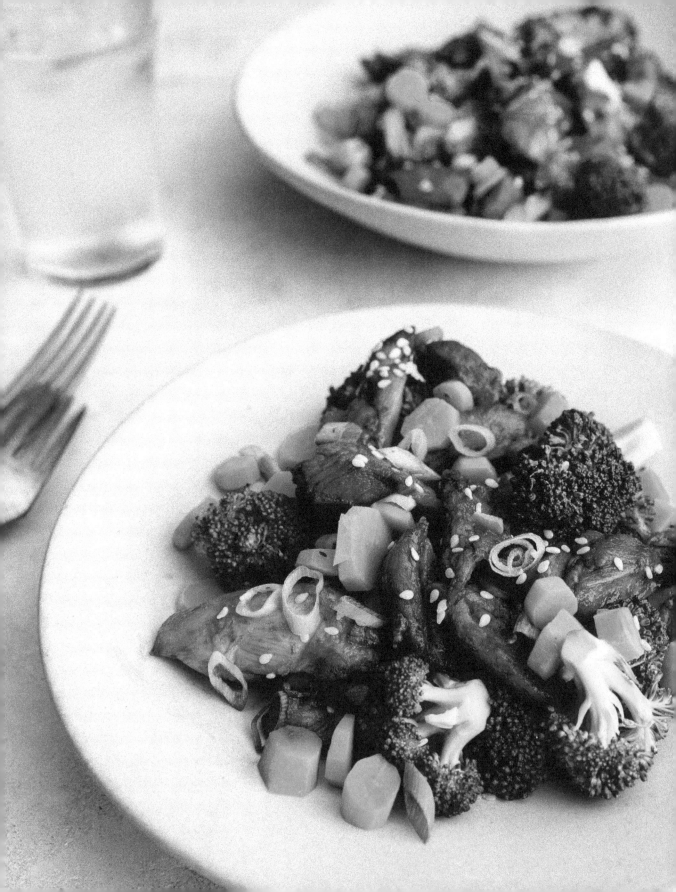

CHAPTER ONE

IBS and the Power of Diet

You probably feel like you are the only one in the world who has a confusing, frustrating, and unpredictable digestive system. Lauren went through this IBS journey herself, so she knows firsthand how complex IBS is.

We now know so much more about IBS and reducing its symptoms than we used to. As IBS specialist dietitians, Lauren and Audrey (Monash-trained) will decode IBS and offer multiple dietary and nondietary evidence-based strategies to support you along the way.

Orange Chicken and Broccoli Bowl, page 147

Symptoms of IBS

IBS looks different for everyone. Maybe you start each day with no symptoms at all, then you look and feel like you are six months pregnant by bedtime. You may have mild discomfort, sharp stabbing pain, or something in between, depending on the day. It could be that you don't leave the house for fear of having an accident or you must know where the bathrooms are everywhere you go. Your bowels may move five times a day or once every five days. Your symptoms could happen daily and then disappear for a month. Either way, IBS can be debilitating.

People with IBS often experience confusing and unpredictable digestive symptoms. The most common symptoms include:

- Bloating (pressure in your abdominal area)
- Distension (when your waistline grows)
- Gas production
- Abdominal pain or discomfort
- Altered bowel movements (diarrhea or constipation)

In addition, reflux, the feeling of incomplete emptying, depression, anxiety, fatigue, difficulty sleeping, and a poorer quality of life can sometimes go hand in hand with IBS. You may experience all or just a few of these, too.

What Is IBS?

Irritable bowel syndrome (IBS) is a functional gut disorder. Although your digestive system is medically healthy, it is not working as well as it could be. No one knows exactly what triggers the onset of IBS, but contracting a gut infection is a common trigger. Stress, anxiety, and depression may increase the chance of someone developing IBS, which often includes a combination of the following main factors:

Abdominal hypersensitivity: People with IBS have more abdominal pain or discomfort. They seem to be very sensitive to things that "stretch" the digestive system, such as a sudden increase in gas production or eating a very large meal.

It could be that your gut is sending too many messages to the brain, which over-stimulates the parts responsible for pain. In addition, stress, anxiety, and depression can complicate matters. We know that the brain-gut connection plays an important role.

Intestinal motility: Another consideration with IBS may be that your intestinal motility is poorly tuned. Therefore, your intestines may push things through too quickly or too slowly. This can lead to diarrhea, constipation, or a confusing mix of both.

Gut dysbiosis: We know that there are differences in the gut microbiota of people with IBS. Although at this stage, science is unsure about what impact this has, we understand that the microorganisms do play a role.

Luckily, this book includes many dietary and nondietary therapies that can help you live without symptoms.

FACTORS THAT WORSEN IBS

There are several things that can make IBS symptoms worse.

FODMAP intolerance: FODMAPs are a group of rapidly fermentable carbohydrates found in a variety of different foods. They are known to trigger symptoms in people with IBS. Following a low-FODMAP diet can help you feel a whole lot better.

Psychological factors: Emotions such as stress, anxiety, and depression can have an impact on your digestive system, as the brain-gut connection is very strong. Some people may find that emotions stimulate the digestive system, leading to urgent diarrhea, while others may find the opposite, leading to days of constipation. Psychological factors can heighten sensitivity of the digestive system and lead to feelings of bloating, abdominal discomfort, and pain.

PMS: The hormones released during PMS can heighten your body's sensitivity to pain. Women also find that their IBS symptoms change or get worse just before their period. Joanna Baker, APD, wrote an excellent article on her website titled, "Does Your Period Make IBS Worse?".

Medications and supplements: Certain medications and supplements can affect the digestive system. Talk to your doctor and pharmacist to make sure that you are on the best regime to improve your medical conditions while minimizing gut symptoms.

Reflux: This is where the acid from the stomach migrates backward up the esophagus. The causes of reflux could be multifactorial. However, the sensations are often mixed with those of IBS.

Food allergies or other intolerances: Some food allergies and intolerances can trigger gut symptoms. Work with an allergist or specialist dietitian if you suspect allergies or intolerances that are not related to FODMAPs. Please note that the commonly available IgG food sensitivity blood test is not supported by research and should not be used to detect food intolerances.

Given that high-FODMAP foods are often huge triggers for people with IBS, we are keen to share our easiest low-FODMAP recipes and a 28-day meal plan to reduce your stress and make food easy again.

TYPES OF IBS

IBS can be classified into four subtypes:

IBS-C (constipation): lumpy or hard, difficult to pass, or infrequent bowel movements

IBS-D (diarrhea): frequent and loose or watery bowel movements

IBS-M (mixed): a mix of both constipation and diarrhea

IBS-U (unclassified): for people who don't fit into any of the other groups

There is a very wide range of normal when it comes to bowel routines. The goal is to have bowel movements that are passed comfortably and are not urgent.

Diagnosing IBS

Unfortunately, IBS can't be diagnosed with a blood test or a breath test. You can't find it with an endoscopy or colonoscopy, either. The path to being diagnosed with IBS can be lengthy, but it must always start by speaking with your doctor.

Thankfully, a set of criteria exists to clinically diagnose IBS based on symptoms. According to the Rome IV Criteria, a diagnosis of IBS requires that patients have recurrent abdominal pain on at least one day per week, on average, during the previous three months that is associated with two or more of the following:

- Defecation

- A change in stool frequency

- A change in stool form or consistency

In addition, it is prudent for your doctor to decide if you should be screened for other conditions such as celiac disease, inflammatory bowel diseases (ulcerative colitis, microscopic colitis, and Crohn's disease), and cancer.

Screening for celiac disease deserves a special mention. For the tests to be accurate, you must consume an adequate amount of gluten for several weeks prior. This is called a gluten challenge. Please note that the IgG food intolerance blood test does not diagnose either celiac disease or IBS.

QUESTIONS TO ASK YOUR DOCTOR

It is always important to involve your doctor when you have digestive symptoms. In preparation for meeting with your doctor, you should keep track of the type, frequency, and severity of your symptoms and when they started. This information will help paint a clearer picture so that the doctor can screen you for the appropriate conditions and advise you on the best types of therapies.

Here are some things to discuss with your doctor if you suspect you have IBS:

- Are there other conditions I should be screened for?

- Could stress be a factor?

- Should I try the low-FODMAP diet?

- Would adding more fiber to my diet help or make it worse?

- Are there other therapies or medications that may help?

Sometimes there are signs that you have something more serious going on. The following are red flags that should be considered by your doctor: the onset of symptoms after the age of 50, blood in your stool, family history of digestive conditions, nocturnal bowel movements, unintended weight loss, recurrent vomiting, progressively severe symptoms, and persistent daily diarrhea.

Managing IBS Through Diet

Diet plays a huge role in reducing IBS symptoms. There are some simple dietary changes that can help. They will differ based on your pattern of symptoms, but here are some general recommendations to get you started.

- Avoid missing meals or leaving long gaps between meals.

- Drink at least 8 cups of water per day.

- Review your fiber intake with a dietitian and increase or decrease as needed.

- Swallow less air by eating slowly and limiting fizzy drinks such as soda and beer.

- Avoid sorbitol (an artificial sweetener found in chewing gum and low-sugar candies) if you experience diarrhea.

- Limit gut irritants such as caffeine and alcohol.

- Be mindful that spicy foods can trigger symptoms for some people.

Sometimes these small changes can have a big impact. However, if this is not enough, the low-FODMAP diet is your best next step. Consider enlisting the help of an experienced dietitian from the Monash FODMAP Dietitians Directory to support you along the way.

Understanding FODMAPs

"FODMAP" is a fun acronym that describes a group of small and hard to digest carbohydrates. Here are the meanings behind the scientific terms, which may bring you back to 10th-grade chemistry class.

F stands for "fermentable." Fermentation is the process in which the microorganisms in your colon eat carbohydrates and produce gas as a by-product. They think of it as a special gift for you.

O stands for "oligosaccharide." "Oligo" means few and "saccharide" refers to sugars. Therefore, an oligosaccharide is a short chain of a few sugar molecules. There are two types of oligosaccharides: fructooligosaccharides (also called "FOS" or "fructans") and galactooligosaccharides (GOS). The main foods in this group include wheat, garlic, onion, kidney beans, baked beans, green peas, pistachios, cashews, and chicory root (inulin).

D stands for "disaccharide." "Di" refers to two, so a disaccharide has two sugar molecules. In this case, the dual sugar is lactose. Lactose is found in varying amounts in some (not all) dairy products. Milk and yogurt contain high amounts of lactose while cheeses and butter contain much less.

M stands for "monosaccharide." "Mono" means one, so a monosaccharide is one single sugar. In this case it's fructose. An excess amount of fructose is found in foods such as apples, pears, mangos, asparagus, artichokes, honey, and processed foods with high-fructose corn syrup.

A stands for "and." That one is easy.

P stands for "polyol." These are sugar alcohols found naturally in foods such as apples, pears, cauliflower, mushrooms, and avocados. They are also added to things like gum, low-sugar candies, and supplements. You can usually spot a polyol on a food label because it ends in "ol." Examples include sorbitol, mannitol, and xylitol.

Why are these little carbohydrates so troublesome for people with IBS? The short answer is that most FODMAPs are poorly digested by everyone. Given that a person with IBS has a very sensitive system, high-FODMAP meals can be problematic. Think of your individual FODMAP load like a cup. You can continue to eat smaller amounts of FODMAPs throughout your day, but once you reach your limit, your cup will spill over. You know what that means, right?

MONASH UNIVERSITY LOW-FODMAP DIET RESOURCES

The low-FODMAP diet is complicated, and it can feel impossibly tricky to find your triggers on your own. Don't despair. The gastroenterology research team at Monash University has a suite of resources to help!

The Monash University FODMAP diet app is a must-have tool that is truly worth using every day. It contains the FODMAP content of more than 800 everyday foods. We recommend downloading the app, as new foods are regularly added. It also goes without saying that you should "follow" everything Monash, like their blog and social media feeds.

In addition, Monash offers a powerful and comprehensive training program for dietitians. They recommend embarking on this diet with the support from an experienced dietitian. Audrey has completed this training. For a list of Monash-trained dietitians worldwide, go to the Monash FODMAP Dietitians Directory on their website.

FODMAP Food Lists

You cannot easily guess which foods contain FODMAPs. The FODMAP content of foods is tested by Monash University and published in the Monash University FODMAP diet app. We have summarized the most common foods here. Refer to the Monash app for the comprehensive list and to get updates. If there is a food that has not been tested by Monash, avoid it during the low-FODMAP diet stage; you can test it later during FODMAP reintroduction (see page 66).

Pay special attention when selecting foods labeled with an asterisk (*), as these can often be made using high-FODMAP ingredients.

Low-FODMAP Foods

These low-FODMAP foods contain either no FODMAPs or a small amount in a usual serving size. Choose these foods most of the time.

GRAIN PRODUCTS

- Bread, made without wheat, rye, or barley*
- Bread, traditionally made with wheat or spelt sourdough*
- Corn chips, plain
- Cornstarch
- Flour, buckwheat
- Flour, corn
- Flour, gluten-free*
- Flour, rice
- Oats, rolled
- Pasta, quinoa, rice, or corn*
- Potato starch
- Rice, brown
- Rice crackers*
- Rice Krispies
- Rice noodles*
- Rice, white
- Tapioca starch

VEGETABLES

- Beans, green
- Bok choy
- Broccoli heads
- Cabbage, green
- Carrots
- Chives
- Cucumbers
- Eggplant
- Kale
- Leeks, green parts only
- Lettuce, all types
- Mushrooms, canned
- Parsnips
- Peppers, red bell
- Potatoes, yellow or red
- Scallions, green parts only
- Spinach
- Squash, kabocha
- Tomatoes

FRUIT

- Banana chips
- Bananas, unripe
- Cantaloupe
- Grapes
- Kiwis
- Lemons
- Limes
- Oranges
- Pineapple
- Raspberries
- Rhubarb
- Strawberries

DAIRY AND NONDAIRY ALTERNATIVES

- Butter
- Cheese, cottage, lactose-free
- Cheese, cream, lactose-free
- Cheese, hard
- Cheese, soy*
- Cream, whipped
- Ice cream, lactose-free*
- Margarine
- Milk, almond
- Milk, lactose-free
- Sour cream, lactose-free
- Yogurt, coconut*
- Yogurt, flavored, lactose-free*
- Yogurt, plain, lactose-free

PROTEIN

- Beef
- Chicken
- Edamame
- Eggs
- Fish, all types
- Macadamia nuts
- Peanuts
- Pork
- Pumpkin seeds
- Shellfish, all types
- Sunflower seeds
- Tofu, firm or extra-firm
- Turkey
- Walnuts

Note: Avoid processed meats that contain high-FODMAP ingredients.

BEVERAGES

- Beer
- Coffee
- Cranberry juice
- Vodka
- Wine, red and white

Note: Coffee and alcohol are gut stimulants or irritants. Limit to 1 serving of each per day.

PANTRY

- Chocolate, dark
- Cocoa
- Mayonnaise*
- Miso
- Mustard*
- Nutritional yeast
- Oils, all types*
- Olives
- Soy sauce
- Spices*
- Sugar, brown
- Sugar, white
- Syrup, brown rice
- Syrup, maple
- Worcestershire sauce
- Vinegar, apple cider
- Vinegar, balsamic
- Vinegar, rice-wine
- Vinegar, white
- Xanthan gum
- Yeast

Moderate-FODMAP Foods

The moderate FODMAPs are foods that have a small serving size limit. As the serving size increases, they will change from low-FODMAP to high-FODMAP. Refer to the Monash University FODMAP diet app for the serving-size limit. These limits are per meal, not per day, so you just need to wait two to three hours before enjoying more of those foods. We have included moderate-FODMAP foods in our recipes in low-FODMAP amounts. Please note that for these recipes, there is information in the FODMAP Tip about eating a low-FODMAP serving size for that meal.

GRAIN PRODUCTS

- Flour, almond
- Oats, quick-cooking

VEGETABLES

- Celery
- Corn on the cob
- Peppers, green bell
- Pumpkin, canned
- Sugar snap peas
- Sweet potato
- Tomato, canned
- Zucchini

FRUIT

- Avocados
- Bananas, ripe
- Blueberries
- Cranberries, dried
- Pomegranate seeds
- Raisins

DAIRY AND NONDAIRY ALTERNATIVES

- Cheese, cottage
- Cheese, cream
- Cheese, ricotta
- Cream
- Coconut milk, canned

PROTEIN

- Almonds
- Beans, black, canned
- Chia seeds
- Chickpeas, canned
- Flaxseed
- Lentils, canned
- Lentils, red, dried

PANTRY

- Chocolate, milk
- Ketchup
- Peanut butter

High-FODMAP Foods

These are some of the most common high-FODMAP foods to avoid during the low-FODMAP diet. It may seem like a daunting list, but there are many low-FODMAP alternatives that you can enjoy.

GRAINS

- Barley
- Bread, wheat as main ingredient
- Flour, coconut
- Flour, soy
- Inulin or chicory root
- Rye

VEGETABLES

- Artichokes, fresh
- Asparagus
- Cauliflower
- Garlic
- Garlic powder
- Leeks, bulb
- Mushrooms, button
- Onions, bulb
- Onion powder
- Peas, green

FRUIT

- Apples
- Cherries
- Dried fruit
- Grapefruit
- Mangoes
- Nectarines
- Peaches
- Pears
- Plums
- Watermelon

DAIRY AND NONDAIRY ALTERNATIVES

- Buttermilk
- Chocolate milk
- Frozen yogurt
- Ice cream
- Kefir
- Milk
- Milk, skim milk powder
- Milk, soy, made from whole soybeans
- Yogurt

Note: Avoid dairy products that contain lactose.

PROTEIN

- Beans, baked
- Beans, kidney
- Beans, navy
- Beans, soy, whole
- Cashews
- Crab meat, imitation (may contain sorbitol)
- Pistachios

PANTRY

- Agave
- Fructose
- Glucose-fructose
- High-fructose corn syrup
- Honey
- Mannitol
- Sorbitol
- Xylitol

Note: Avoid sauces and dressings that contain high-FODMAP ingredients unless they have specifically been okayed by Monash.

BEVERAGES

- Juice, most types
- Tea, fennel
- Tea, chamomile

Why Do FODMAPs Trigger IBS Symptoms in Some People?

FODMAPs have several ways of triggering symptoms. Oligosaccharides are poorly absorbed in the small intestine by everyone. Once they reach your colon, they become a delectable feast for the bacteria that live there. The bacteria thank you in spades by producing generous quantities of gas.

Fructose and polyols are naturally slowly absorbed in the small intestine. As they move along, they hold on to water. When this watery FODMAP-filled mix flows into the colon, they are also enthusiastically enjoyed by the gut bacteria.

Lactose is the sugar found in dairy products. In order for lactose to be absorbed in the small intestine, it needs to be split into two smaller sugars (glucose and galactose) by the lactase enzyme. However, some people don't make enough of the lactase enzyme. Similar to fructose and polyols, some lactose may remain in the small intestine, where it attracts water and then flows into the colon. For the bacteria, it's like Free Slurpee Day at the 7-Eleven!

These processes, in combination with a system that is already hypersensitive, can lead to gas, bloating, pain or discomfort, and altered bowel movements for people with IBS.

The Low-FODMAP Diet for IBS

The low-FODMAP diet is a medical diet (not a weight-loss diet) designed to reduce your symptoms and identify food triggers in three stages. By reducing the amount of FODMAPs temporarily, most people with IBS will feel significantly better.

Step 1: Low-FODMAP diet. Replace high-FODMAP foods with low-FODMAP foods to reduce your overall FODMAP intake. In the Monash app, choose the green-light servings most of the time and avoid the red-light servings. This phase lasts for two to six weeks, depending on your symptom improvement.

Step 2: FODMAP reintroduction. Systematically test high-FODMAP foods, one FODMAP group at a time, over three days while increasing the serving size to discover which FODMAP groups trigger symptoms.

Step 3: FODMAP personalization. Expand your diet by eating foods from the groups that didn't cause you any symptoms. You will still need to limit foods that triggered symptoms. Retest them in a few weeks to see if your tolerance has improved.

THE LOW-FODMAP DIET IS HELPFUL FOR OTHER CONDITIONS, TOO

Research shows that a trial of the low-FODMAP diet can be helpful for people who have other health conditions if they also experience ongoing digestive symptoms.

Celiac disease: When people with celiac experience gut symptoms despite following a strict gluten-free diet, they may benefit from a trial of the low-FODMAP diet.

Inflammatory bowel diseases: The low-FODMAP diet can be helpful for people with inflammatory bowel disease who experience digestive symptoms not associated with a flare-up.

Endometriosis: The low-FODMAP diet can help reduce abdominal pain among women with endometriosis.

Childhood and adolescent IBS: A low-FODMAP diet can be used for children and adolescents with IBS. To support their needs for growth and development while on a restrictive diet, it is highly recommended that you work with an experienced dietitian and follow the diet for the shortest length of time needed to reduce symptoms.

SIBO: The low-FODMAP diet may help with the management of small intestinal bacterial overgrowth (SIBO), though research is limited.

Other Treatments for IBS

There are several additional strategies supported by medical research that you can use to reduce IBS symptoms. The strategy you choose will depend on your symptoms.

Psychological therapies: Gut-directed hypnotherapy and cognitive behavior therapy, when led by a registered psychologist, are very effective for helping with IBS.

Soluble fiber supplement: A soluble fiber supplement may help with diarrhea and constipation. Of the many supplements available, psyllium husk and partially hydrolyzed guar gum (PHGG) are the most widely studied. Start with a small amount, increase over a week, and make sure you drink enough water. Be aware that fiber supplements can sometimes increase gas production. Avoid products that contain inulin, FOS, wheat bran, or other high-FODMAP ingredients.

Therapies for constipation: You have a few great options. There are compounds in coffee that stimulate your colon. A footstool under your feet while on the toilet helps position you for a satisfying bowel movement. Polyethylene glycol (PEG) is a safe and effective laxative. PEG is not habit-forming and doesn't contribute to additional gas production. Magnesium citrate can help soften bowel movements. It is best to talk to a pharmacist about the latter two options.

Digestive enzymes: The lactase enzyme can help partially digest lactose for people with lactose intolerance. The alpha galactosidase enzyme may reduce gas and bloating from eating foods high in galactooligosaccharides. Avoid products with polyol sweeteners.

Enteric-coated peppermint: Peppermint oil can help with abdominal pain and spasms. It needs to be enteric-coated, so it bypasses the stomach and goes to work on the small intestine. It should be avoided if you experience reflux.

Probiotics: Probiotics may help with IBS; however, improvements are often mild. Choose one with research to match your symptoms (www.usprobioticguide.com). Avoid probiotics with high-FODMAP ingredients. Take them daily, and watch for improvements over a four-week period.

Pharmaceuticals: There are several effective medications for IBS that are worth talking to your doctor about, such as antidiarrheals, laxatives, antispasmodics, antibiotics, and antidepressants (used for pain).

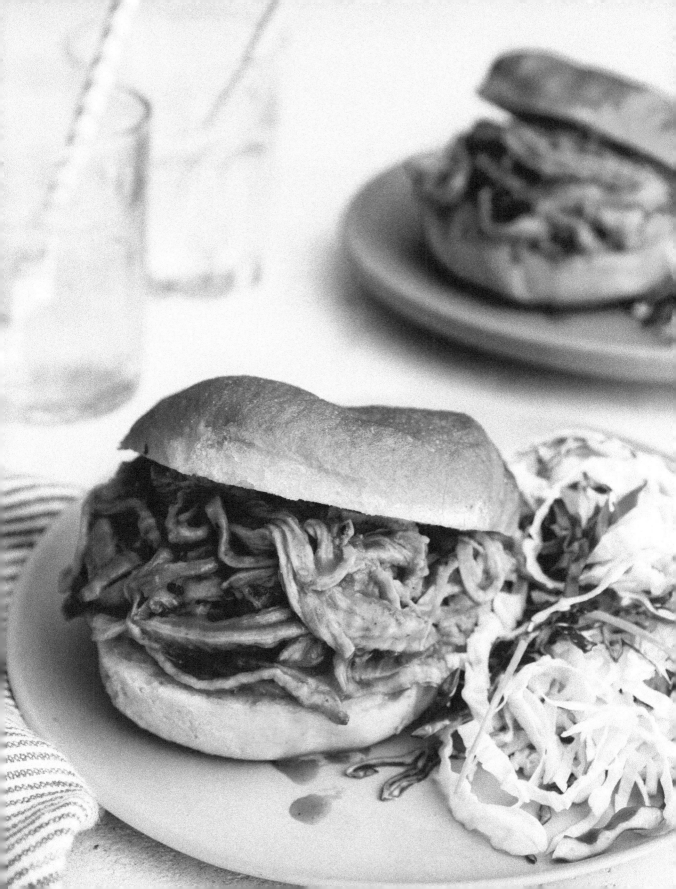

CHAPTER TWO

Preparing for the Weeks Ahead

It is with excitement and anticipation that we will walk beside you on this path over the next few weeks. We are very proud that you are here.

But is there something holding you back? A vacation? A family to feed? A lack of time? There's no benefit to waiting. This diet is not about being perfect or starting at the perfect time. Your goal is to reduce your overall FODMAP intake enough to relieve your symptoms. That doesn't require perfection.

Our recipes are easy, with a minimal number of simple ingredients. And did we mention delicious? Our dinners can feed your whole family, so you don't have to make multiple meals. Your family members without IBS can simply add or substitute high-FODMAP alternatives such as wheat bread, wheat pasta, and garlic.

Our meal plans are simple, so you don't have to think about what to serve for a whole month. We recommend cooking your food at home most of the time, which is good for everyone regardless of whether you have IBS. You gain health, spend less money, and feel better. Lucky you!

Barbecue Pulled Pork, page 151

Getting the Most Out of Your Meal Plan

While writing this book, we have absolutely loved putting our heads together to share the best tips we've picked up from coaching thousands of people on the low-FODMAP diet. Here are the four main steps that we think you should start with.

STEP 1: READ NUTRITION LABELS LIKE A PRO

Knowing what is in your food is paramount to your success. You will get into the habit of reading the label of everything that goes down the hatch, including food, beverages, gum, and even supplements. Please note that the foods listed with an asterisk (*) have a very small acceptable serving size according to the Monash app. However, it is hard to know how much of those ingredients are in packaged foods. For example, molasses has a small acceptable serving size, but it is difficult to guess whether a cookie containing molasses would be low-FODMAP. For now, we recommend avoiding packaged foods that contain ingredients listed on page 25 unless they have been tested by Monash or are certified as low-FODMAP.

TIP: Take a photo of this list, so you can refer to it as needed.

COMMON HIGH-FODMAP INGREDIENTS

SWEETENERS

- Agave*
- Apple juice
- Coconut sugar*
- Fructose
- Fruit juice
- Fruit juice concentrate
- Glucose-fructose
- Golden syrup*
- High-fructose corn syrup
- Honey*
- Isomalt
- Mannitol
- Molasses*
- Pear juice
- Polydextrose
- Sorbitol
- Xylitol

FLAVORINGS

- Garlic
- Garlic powder
- Garlic salt
- Onion powder
- Onions
- Onion salt

DAIRY

- Buttermilk
- Kefir
- Lactose
- Milk
- Milk, condensed
- Milk, skim, powder
- Milk solids
- Modified milk ingredients
- Whey protein concentrate

FLOURS, GRAINS, NUTS, AND PULSES

- Amaranth
- Barley
- Bulgur
- Cashews
- Couscous
- Flour, chickpea
- Flour, coconut
- Flour, lentil
- Kamut
- Pistachios
- Rye
- Semolina
- Soybeans, whole
- Soy flours
- Textured vegetable protein (TVP)
- Wheat*
- Whole soybeans

OTHER ADDITIVES

- Chicory root
- Fructooligosaccharides (FOS)
- Inulin
- VitaFiber

The following foods can be tricky because they may or may not include high-FODMAPs. Here's our advice on finding the low-FODMAP choices. You can also refer to the Low-FODMAP Resources (page 197) and the Monash app for companies that sell certified low-FODMAP foods.

Bananas: The FODMAP content of bananas increases as they ripen. A medium unripe banana is low-FODMAP, but a ripe banana with brown spots is not; you should limit yourself to one-third of a fully ripe banana. The color of the peel of an unripe banana is a combination of yellow and green. Storing bananas in the refrigerator or freezer stops the ripening process. Don't forget to label your frozen bananas as either ripe or unripe.

Beverages: Many sugar-sweetened beverages are made with high-fructose corn syrup or concentrated fruit juice, so they should be avoided for now. Most diet sodas are low-FODMAP; however, we recommend that you hydrate with water most of the time. Flavored sparkling waters with 0 grams of carbohydrates on the nutrition label are another low-FODMAP option. But be aware that when you swallow bubbles, they have to make their exit by going either up or down.

Bread: You have two main choices for bread. Traditional sourdough bread made from wheat or spelt is lower in FODMAPs, as the traditional sourdough process breaks down the fructans when the bread is leavened for more than 12 hours. Avoid sourdough bread that contains high-FODMAP ingredients, such as barley or rye (see page 25), and check the Monash app for the low-FODMAP serving size. Your second option is gluten-free bread. Choose the brands made with low-FODMAP flours (see page 28). In addition, read the ingredient list very carefully, and avoid bread made with high-FODMAP ingredients, such as inulin or high-fructose corn syrup.

Condiments: When a condiment has not been tested by Monash, avoid it if it contains onions, garlic, or other high-FODMAP ingredients. Ketchup, Worcestershire sauce, soy sauce, and Sriracha were tested by Monash and were found to have a small low-FODMAP serving size, despite the fact that they contain high-FODMAP ingredients.

Crackers: Rice crackers and saltines are low-FODMAP but have serving size limits. Refer to the Monash app for the amounts. Gluten-free crackers may also be low-FODMAP, but avoid the ones with high-FODMAP ingredients.

Dairy: The lactose content of dairy varies depending on the type. Butter is naturally very low in lactose. Cheeses are naturally low in lactose with some exceptions like ricotta, cream cheese, and cottage cheese. You will need to limit your serving size to 1 to 2 tablespoons per meal or choose the lactose-free versions. Milk, yogurt, and ice cream are much higher in lactose, so you should choose the lactose-free versions. However, be watchful because not all lactose-free dairy products are low-FODMAP. Avoid the ones that contain high-FODMAP ingredients such as high-FODMAP fruits or sweeteners.

Deli meat: Choose deli meats that exclude onions, garlic, and high-FODMAP sweeteners.

Flour: Common low-FODMAP flours include rice, buckwheat, corn, millet, potato, tapioca, sorghum, teff, and quinoa. Lauren commonly uses almond flour and oat flour, which both have small low-FODMAP serving sizes. Read the ingredient list carefully and avoid flours with high-FODMAP ingredients such as chickpea, coconut, and soy (see page 25). Many flour blends contain xanthan gum or guar gum, which are both low-FODMAP, to help with texture.

Scallions, leeks, and chives: The green leaves of scallions, leeks, and chives are low-FODMAP. We use them generously in our recipes to replace the onion bulb. Use only the parts that are dark green, not the parts that become lighter in color. Chives are green throughout, so you don't have to discard any part of them. Leeks and chives freeze well.

Nondairy beverages: Almond milk is low-FODMAP. Other nondairy beverages have serving size limits or are high-FODMAP. Refer to the Monash app for more information.

Pasta: Choose pasta that is made from rice, corn, quinoa, or other low-FODMAP grains. Read the ingredient list carefully, and avoid pasta made with high-FODMAP ingredients (see page 25).

Soup broth: When choosing vegetable, chicken, or beef broth, avoid the brands with onion, garlic, and other high-FODMAP ingredients. We have noticed that finding low-FODMAP vegetable broth is more difficult than finding low-FODMAP chicken or beef broth, which is why we included our recipe for Nourishing Vegetable Broth (page 178). You can also find certified low-FODMAP brands in the Monash Low-FODMAP App.

Spices: Avoid spice mixes that contain onions or garlic, such as steak seasoning or chili powder.

Tea: Rooibos, green, or peppermint teas are low-FODMAP, while black tea has limits. Avoid teas that contain chicory root, high-FODMAP fruits, chamomile, or fennel.

STEP 3: CREATE YOUR LOW-FODMAP KITCHEN

Now it's time to move into your kitchen and grab a permanent marker. In your refrigerator, set aside or give away your lactose-containing dairy, as it will likely expire over the next few weeks. Review the ingredient lists of your condiments, jams, deli meats, and other refrigerator items. Write a happy face on the ones that are low-FODMAP. In your pantry, create a low-FODMAP space. Scan the ingredient lists of crackers, cookies, cereals, canned goods, pastas, and teas. Draw a happy face on the ones that are low-FODMAP, and start to populate your new space. You'll have a few more things to add after your trip to the grocery store.

STEP 4: TAKE 10 MINUTES TO PLAN YOUR WEEK

Meal planning is not an insurmountable task. With our weekly meal plans and a little practice, you'll be done in 10 minutes each week, tops. Record your meals in the most convenient place, such as your phone calendar or kitchen calendar, or snap a photo of it. Use the grocery lists we provide, and record any additional ingredients you will need. Then go shopping, or order your groceries online. Be sure to give yourself a little extra time in the grocery store to apply your new label-reading skills.

Stock Your Pantry

Having a well-stocked pantry will make your month much easier. You don't need to have every single ingredient at all times. Check your personalized grocery list each week to fill in the items you need. You may want to buy some ingredients like spices and flours in bulk to save a few dollars where you can.

Any ingredient with an asterisk (*) beside it indicates that you should read labels to check for any high-FODMAP ingredients (see page 25).

GRAINS

Although wheat is high-FODMAP, don't worry, there are plenty of low-FODMAP grains you can enjoy. Be aware that gluten-free does not necessarily mean low-FODMAP. Read every ingredient list carefully, and watch for high-FODMAP ingredients.

- Bread crumbs*
- Corn tortillas*
- Crackers*
- Oats, rolled
- Pasta, quinoa, rice, or corn*
- Quinoa
- Rice
- Rice cereal
- Rice crackers*
- Rice noodles

OIL, VINEGAR, SPICES, AND WINE

The spices, oils, and vinegars in your pantry will help make each meal delicious, and white cooking wine will add a splash of flavor. Make sure to store your oils in a dark place away from sources of heat to help them stay fresh.

- Anchovy paste*
- Cooking spray, nonstick
- Cooking wine, white
- Herbs, dried (basil, bay leaves, chipotle chile powder or ancho chile powder, cinnamon, cumin, ginger, Italian seasoning, lemon-pepper seasoning, oregano, smoked paprika, turmeric)*
- Mustard, dry
- Nutritional yeast
- Peppercorns
- Oil, coconut
- Oil, olive, extra-virgin
- Oil, sesame
- Salt
- Tabasco sauce
- Vinegar (apple cider, balsamic, red-wine, rice, white)

NUTS AND SEEDS

Nuts and seeds are nutritional powerhouses, packed with heart-healthy fats, protein, and fiber. We recommend storing them in the freezer to help prevent them from going rancid.

- Almond butter
- Almonds
- Chia seeds
- Flaxseed
- Peanut butter
- Peanuts
- Pumpkin seeds (pepitas)
- Sunflower seeds
- Walnuts

BAKING

It can feel next to impossible to find low-FODMAP baked goods in bakeries. Low-FODMAP baking may seem intimidating, but our recipes are simple and taste just as good (if not better!) than the original versions.

- Almond flour
- Baking powder
- Baking soda
- Chocolate chips, semisweet
- Cocoa powder
- Coconut, shredded, unsweetened
- Cornstarch
- Cranberries, dried*
- Flour, glutinous or sweet rice (for crêpes)
- Flour blend, low-FODMAP
- Maple syrup
- Sugar, brown and white
- Vanilla extract

CANNED OR JARRED

It's smart to stock up on canned and jarred foods during sales. Once you open a can, transfer any leftover food to a reusable container, and place in the refrigerator.

- Beans, black, canned
- Chicken broth*
- Chickpeas, canned
- Ketchup
- Lentils, canned
- Lentils, red, dried
- Mayonnaise*
- Mushrooms, canned
- Mustard*
- Olives, Kalamata, pitted
- Peppers, jalapeño*
- Strained
- Pickles*
- Pineapple, canned
- Roasted red peppers, jarred
- Soy sauce
- Sriracha
- Tomatoes, strained of skins and seeds (passata)*
- Tomatoes, sun-dried, jarred
- Tomato juice
- Tomato paste
- Tomato sauce*
- Tuna, canned

Essential Equipment

We are low-key when it comes to kitchen appliances. Neither of us have specialized cooking equipment in our kitchens, so our recipes use just the basics.

Pots and pans: You will need an assortment of pots and pans. We recommend having a small pot, a medium pot, a large soup pot, and a large skillet, preferably nonstick.

Sheet pans: Sheet pans are great for making cookies, sheet pan meals, and roasted vegetables.

Muffin tin: A muffin tin is used to make the Banana-Carrot Muffins (page 172), Banana–Chocolate Chip Oatmeal Bites (page 85), and "Rise and Shine" Egg Muffins (page 74). Tins can also be used for freezing foods in small portions (e.g., sauces, cooked lentils).

Baking dish: A standard glass 8-inch square baking dish is versatile and can be used for a variety of our dishes. We also use a larger 9-by-13-inch baking dish for a few recipes.

Knives and a knife sharpener: These are the three types of knives that we use most. In addition, don't forget that a sharp knife is a cook's best friend. If you don't have a knife sharpener, don't be intimidated. Buy one—it is money well spent. Knives are relatively easy to sharpen (just perform a search online). You'll be slicing tomatoes like a pro in no time.

- Paring knife: useful for peeling fruits and vegetables
- Chef's knife: an all-purpose knife for cutting all types of food
- Serrated knife: ideal for cutting bread

Cutting board with nonstick feet: There is nothing worse than cutting on a board that slides all over the counter. Audrey loves the cutting boards with rubber feet on the corners to hold the cutting board in place.

Box grater and zester: A grater is needed for the cheese recipes and to grate the sweet potato for the Sweet Potato Quinoa Cakes (page 97). A good rasp can help add zest to your meals.

Slow cooker or electric pressure cooker: You certainly don't need both. But it would be nice to have one or the other. You'll thank us on the day you make slow-roasted Barbecue Pulled Pork (page 151) or the Slow Cooker Beef Stew (page 157). Imagine walking into the house after a long day's work to a dinner that literally cooked itself. You'll feel so spoiled.

Rice cooker: Rice cookers are super convenient for making both rice and quinoa. You add the ingredients, then walk away. Cookers automatically stop cooking, so your rice and quinoa are perfect every time.

Blender: A blender is a necessity if you like smoothies. You don't have to spend a fortune on a blender; you can buy a good-quality one on Amazon for less than $100. They are also splendid for emulsifying the Caesar Vinaigrette (page 188) or blending a quick pesto. An alternative is an immersion blender, which is also very convenient for soups.

Jars and containers: Audrey always has a revolving door of salad dressing shakers filled with homemade dressings in her refrigerator. They take up very little space, don't dribble down the side, and are available on Amazon or at the grocery store. Mason jars are ideal for making a large batch of Cajun seasoning to last you for the month. Extra Mason jars can also be used for overnight oats to take on the go.

Nesting lunch and snack containers: It is a great idea for everyone to bring healthy food with them for snacks throughout the day. If you are on a special diet, it is absolutely essential. You will need to make sure that you have enough containers because you wouldn't want that to hold you back. The nesting part is not essential; however, if you are in the market, it is worthwhile to get a few that fit together and a few of different sizes.

Kitchen scale: There are several moderate-FODMAP foods that have weight limits in the Monash app. Using a kitchen scale can help you measure the right amount without going over or under. You can find a good scale for less than $30.

Parchment paper: Most people don't enjoy scraping crusty food off pans, which is why parchment paper was invented. We like to use parchment paper as often as possible. Fish in a Bag (page 139) is made using parchment paper and kitchen staples.

Can opener: Canned foods can be cost effective and convenient, as long as you have a good can opener.

Tips and Tricks to Make Your Day Easier

We can all think of things we'd rather do instead of preparing food and washing dishes. Here are some tips and tricks to help reduce the time spent doing both, avoid take-out temptation, reduce food waste, and fill your kitchen with healthy food.

Review your meal plan, and shop once a week. Our meal plans are designed for you to shop for groceries once a week, but you can shop more frequently if that is convenient. You may find that shopping online and getting your groceries delivered means that you stick to the foods on your list, avoid high-FODMAP temptations, and save money and time.

Make extra dinner for lunch the next day. Once you are done eating dinner, pack up your lunch right away. You may even squeeze two lunches out of the deal.

Double the recipes, and store them in the freezer. The freezer is a meal prepper's best friend. Freezers make healthy eating much easier. Why cook a recipe multiple times and make tons of dirty dishes when you could make a large batch and freeze extras for later? Freezing helps preserve freshness and nutrients in food. Always label everything with a low-FODMAP name and date before putting it in the freezer. We like to keep a permanent marker in our box of freezer bags, so it doesn't get lost or borrowed.

Buy prewashed vegetables. Prewashed vegetables like salad greens, coleslaw mix, baby carrots, cherry tomatoes, baby cucumbers, and green beans will save you a lot of time. Everyone in your household will likely eat more vegetables if they are washed and ready.

Prepare a container of mixed vegetables. Certain vegetables, such as baby carrots, cherry tomatoes, baby cucumbers, and baby peppers, will last for several days in the refrigerator. Don't slice the cucumbers and peppers, as they will get slimy.

Freeze extra foods. Your freezer can also be a great tool to help reduce food waste and save money. Always remember to clearly label everything you put in your freezer. Here are the foods we most commonly freeze.

- *Chopped leek greens and chives:* Clean and chop the dark green parts only. Freeze in a labeled freezer bag. When you are ready to use them, simply give the bag a shake to break up the bits, then pour them into your pan or pot. One cup of leeks is roughly equivalent to one medium onion.

- *Greens:* Green leafy vegetables, like spinach, baby kale, and chard, can be placed in a freezer bag and thrown in the freezer. We don't like to pass up opportunities to add greens to smoothies and soups.

- *Tomato sauce, juice, and paste:* Some recipes might require only half a can of tomatoes. If you pour the extra into a freezer bag and let it freeze flat, then it is easy to break off small pieces later.

- *Produce with a small low-FODMAP serving size:* Celery and avocado are two foods that have a small serving size and freeze well. Given that there is a small window of time to enjoy avocado, you may need to freeze it before it expires. To freeze an avocado, mash it with lemon or lime juice and spoon it into ice cube trays or a freezer bag.

- *Chickpeas, black beans, and lentils:* Given that the serving size of these legumes is small, you likely won't use the whole can at one time. They freeze exceptionally well in a freezer bag.

- *Bananas:* Unripe bananas can be frozen to keep them low-FODMAP and stop them from ripening further. Peel them, and put them in a freezer bag. Slice before freezing if using for smoothies, since it's easier on your blender. Dark brown ripe bananas can be frozen and used for baking; one-third of a brown banana is low-FODMAP. Add them to a separate bag labeled as "ripe bananas."

- *Bread:* You can prevent bread from going stale by slicing and freezing. Press out any air in the freezer bag before placing it in the freezer. When you are ready to eat a slice, toast it or reheat it in a microwave. Frozen bread will stay fresh-tasting for a few months.

- *Canned coconut milk:* Freeze in small containers or ice cube trays.

- *Wine, lemon juice, or lime juice:* You can freeze wine, lemon juice, and lime juice in a labeled freezer bag. Let it freeze flat, then break off small pieces as needed. You can also use an ice cube tray for this purpose.

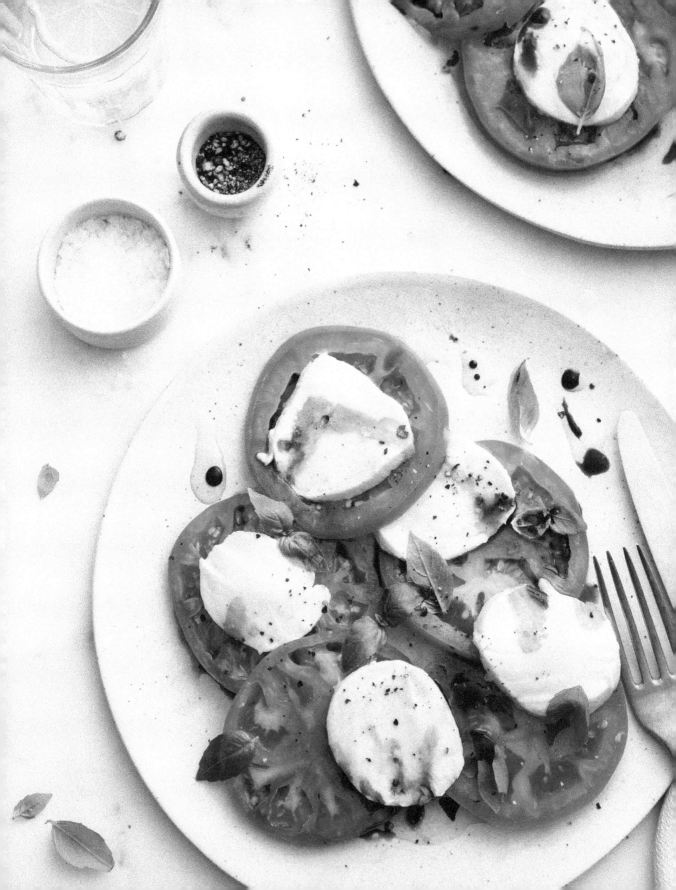

CHAPTER THREE

The 28-Day Meal Plan

Here are your next 28 days of low-FODMAP recipes. Each week includes a meal plan with a grocery list and preparation tips. The amounts in the shopping list are for one person, so you can increase them if you are cooking for more than just yourself.

These handy tips will help you these next four weeks:

- **Download the Monash University FODMAP diet app.**

- **Take pictures of each main meal (or record them in your phone or kitchen calendar), the grocery lists so you can have them with you at the store, and the list of Common High-FODMAP Ingredients (page 25).**

- **Really keen on a specific recipe? Double it and have it instead of another recipe.**

- **The vegetables and fruits used for snacks and lunches are carrots, cucumber, red bell peppers, strawberries, grapes, and oranges. They can be interchanged at any time.**

Caprese Salad, page 93

Week One

It's your first week, and you are feeling a bit nervous and overwhelmed. Take a deep breath—you can do this. Spend a few minutes planning to make sure that you have plenty of delicious low-FODMAP options available throughout your day to keep you satisfied and happy till dinner. Avoid skipping lunch or getting overly hungry, as you want to prevent cravings and feeling deprived. You don't have to do this alone. There are plenty of Monash FODMAP-trained dietitians (see Resources on page 197 for more information).

RATE YOUR SYMPTOMS

Record your baseline symptoms. Use a scale of 1 to 10 (1 is low, 10 is high) and the Bristol Stool Chart to record your bowel movements.

BLOATING	
GAS PRODUCTION	
ABDOMINAL PAIN OR DISCOMFORT	
BOWEL MOVEMENTS	

PREPARATION TIPS

Cook and Store

- Hard-boil 4 eggs
- Cook ⅓ cup quinoa

Make Ahead

- Banana–Chocolate Chip Oatmeal Bites (page 85)
- "Rise and Shine" Egg Muffins (page 74)
- Trail Mix (page 160)
- Maple–Balsamic Vinegar Dressing (page 181)

Freeze

- 8 Banana–Chocolate Chip Oatmeal Bites
- 8 "Rise and Shine" Egg Muffins

PREPARATION NOTES

For the following recipes this week, you will make only a portion of the recipe as follows:

- ½ recipe Tuna Melt (page 132)
- ½ recipe Salmon with Basil-Caper Pesto (page 134)
- ⅓ recipe Greek Quinoa Salad (page 96)
- ½ recipe Prosciutto-Wrapped Chicken (page 145)
- ½ recipe Sheet Pan Steak and Potatoes (page 152)
- ½ recipe Tofu Noodle Bowl (page 114)
- ½ recipe Orange Chicken and Broccoli Bowl (page 147)
- ¼ recipe Bell Pepper Mini Pizzas (page 108)
- ¼ recipe Pomegranate, Poppy Seed, and Spinach Salad (page 102)

WEEK ONE MENU AT A GLANCE

	BREAKFAST	SNACK	LUNCH
M	2 Banana–Chocolate Chip Oatmeal Bites (page 85)	Rice crackers and peanut butter	Curry Egg Salad Sandwich (page 110) with cucumber slices
T	Vanilla-Maple Overnight Oats (page 80) and an orange	Leftover Banana–Chocolate Chip Oatmeal Bite (page 85)	Leftover Salmon with Basil-Caper Pesto (page 134) with rice; green salad with Maple–Balsamic Vinegar Dressing (page 181)
W	Oatmeal Cookie Smoothie (page 78)	Boiled egg and mozzarella slice	Leftover Greek Quinoa Salad (page 96) and leftover Chive-Rubbed Chicken (page 143)
T	2 "Rise and Shine" Egg Muffins (page 74)	Yogurt with strawberries	Leftover Prosciutto-Wrapped Chicken (page 145) and Caprese Salad (page 93)
F	Peanut butter on low-FODMAP toast and an orange	Leftover "Rise and Shine" Egg Muffin (page 74)	Leftover Sheet Pan Steak and Potatoes (page 152)
S	Denver-Style Omelet (page 86) with low-FODMAP toast	Rice crackers with peanut butter	Tuna Melt (page 132) and red bell pepper slices
S	Banana Egg Pancakes (page 87) with peanut butter and chocolate chips	Leftover "Rise and Shine" Egg Muffin (page 74)	Snack plate with ¼ cup Roasted Red Pepper Hummus (page 163), mozzarella slices, cucumber, carrots, and rice crackers

SNACK	DINNER	NOTES
Yogurt and strawberries	Salmon with Basil-Caper Pesto (page 134) with rice; spinach salad with Maple–Balsamic Vinegar Dressing (page 181)	
Mozzarella slice and grapes	Greek Quinoa Salad (page 96) with Chive-Rubbed Chicken (page 143)	
Leftover Banana–Chocolate Chip Oatmeal Bite (page 85)	Prosciutto-Wrapped Chicken (page 145) and Caprese Salad (page 93)	
Trail Mix (page 160)	Sheet Pan Steak and Potatoes (page 152)	
Yogurt with strawberries	Tofu Noodle Bowl (page 114)	
Boiled egg and an orange	Orange Chicken and Broccoli Bowl (page 147)	
Yogurt with grapes	Bell Pepper Mini Pizzas (page 108) with Pomegranate, Poppy Seed, and Spinach Salad (page 102)	

SHOPPING LIST

Canned and bottled items

- Capers, 1 (3-ounce) jar
- Chickpeas, 1 (15½-ounce) can
- Mayonnaise, 1 (8-ounce) jar*
- Mustard, Dijon, smooth, 1 (8-ounce) jar
- Olives, black, 1 (6-ounce) can
- Pickles,* 1 (16-ounce) jar (optional)
- Roasted red peppers, 1 (8-ounce) jar
- Soy sauce, 1 (10-ounce) bottle
- Tahini, 1 (11-ounce) can
- Tomato sauce, 1 (8-ounce) can
- Tuna, water-packed, 1 (6-ounce) can

Dairy and eggs

- Butter (½ pound)
- Cheese, bocconcini (4 ounces)
- Cheese, Cheddar, shredded (⅓ cup)
- Cheese, feta, crumbled (⅓ cup)
- Cheese, goat, crumbled (⅛ cup)
- Cheese, mozzarella (8 ounces)
- Cheese, Parmesan, grated (½ cup)
- Eggs (20)
- Milk, lactose-free or almond (½ gallon)
- Yogurt, plain, lactose-free (16 ounces)

Meat

- Chicken, boneless, skinless breasts (2)
- Chicken, boneless, thighs (12 ounces)
- Prosciutto, sliced (2 ounces)
- Rib eye steak (8 ounces)
- Salmon, 1 (4- to 6-ounce) fillet
- Smoked ham, diced (1½ ounces)

Pantry items

- Almond butter
- Baking powder
- Banana chips
- Basil, dried
- Bay leaves
- Bread*
- Cereal, Crispix
- Chia seeds
- Chives, dried
- Chocolate chips

- Cinnamon, ground
- Cranberries, dried
- Curry powder*
- Maple syrup
- Nonstick cooking spray
- Nutmeg, ground (optional)
- Nutritional yeast
- Oats, rolled
- Oil, olive, extra-virgin
- Oil, sesame
- Oregano, dried
- Peanut butter
- Peanuts
- Peppercorns, black
- Poppy seeds
- Quinoa
- Rice crackers*
- Rice, long-grain
- Rice noodles, thin

- Salt
- Sesame seeds
- Sugar, brown
- Sugar, white
- Vanilla extract
- Vinegar, balsamic
- Vinegar, rice-wine
- Vinegar, white
- Walnuts

Produce

- Bananas, unripe (4)
- Basil, fresh (2 bunches)
- Bell pepper, green (1)
- Bell peppers, red (4)
- Broccoli (1 head)
- Carrots, medium (8)
- Cucumber (1)
- Grapes (12 ounces)
- Kale (1 bunch)

- Lemons (3)
- Mushrooms, oyster (4 ounces)
- Onion, small (1)
- Oranges (3)
- Parsley (1 bunch)
- Pomegranate (1)
- Potatoes, yellow or red, medium (2)
- Scallions (4 bunches)
- Spinach, baby (6 ounces)
- Strawberries, fresh or frozen (1½ pounds)
- Tomatoes (5)
- Tomatoes, cherry (10 ounces)

Other

- Tofu, extra-firm, 1 (14-ounce) package

*Read the ingredient list, and avoid products with high-FODMAP ingredients.

Week Two

Congratulations—you have one week under your belt. For week two, planning is still your top priority. Review your meal plan, and make your list before rushing off to the grocery store. It doesn't matter if your first week wasn't perfect. Your main goal is to learn the diet and reduce your overall FODMAP intake. Give yourself a pat on the back, and don't forget that you can find a Monash FODMAP-trained dietitian in the Resources section (page 197).

RATE YOUR SYMPTOMS

Some people notice a difference right away; others may notice a difference over the course of a few weeks. Everyone is different. Rate your symptoms using a scale of 1 to 10 (1 is low, 10 is high) and the Bristol Stool Chart to record your bowel movements.

BLOATING	
GAS PRODUCTION	
ABDOMINAL PAIN OR DISCOMFORT	
BOWEL MOVEMENTS	

Make Ahead

- Cajun Spice Mix (page 186)
- Peanut Butter Power Balls (page 168)
- Sunshine Granola (page 72)
- ½ recipe Strawberry-Lemon Chia Seed Jam (page 183)

- ½ recipe Carrot-Ginger Soup (page 90)
- Sweet Barbecue Sauce (page 176)
- Goddess Dressing (page 179)

Freeze

- 20 Peanut Butter Power Balls

Plan Ahead

- Wednesday morning: Prepare the Barbecue Pulled Pork (page 151) in the slow cooker or Instant Pot®.

PREPARATION NOTES

For the following recipes this week, you will make only a portion of the recipe as follows:

- ½ recipe Spaghetti Bolognese (page 154)
- ½ recipe Canadian Maple Salmon (page 131)
- ½ recipe Sheet Pan Chicken and Vegetables (page 148)
- ½ recipe Broccoli and Cheese Frittata (page 109)
- ¼ recipe Turkey Burgers (page 149)

- ½ recipe Cajun-Spiced Root Vegetable Fries (page 103)
- ½ recipe Lentil Shepherd's Pie (page 119)
- ½ recipe Strawberry-Lemon Chia Seed Jam (page 183)
- ½ recipe Carrot-Ginger Soup (page 90)

WEEK TWO MENU AT A GLANCE

	BREAKFAST	SNACK	LUNCH
M	Sunshine Granola (page 72) with yogurt and Strawberry-Lemon Chia Seed Jam (page 183)	Leftover Roasted Red Pepper Hummus (page 163) and cucumber	Leftover Orange Chicken and Broccoli Bowl (page 147)
T	Peanut Butter and Chocolate Smoothie (page 76)	Leftover Banana–Chocolate Chip Oatmeal Bite (page 85)	Leftover Spaghetti Bolognese (page 154) with Caesar Salad (page 98)
W	2 leftover "Rise and Shine" Egg Muffins (page 74)	Leftover Sunshine Granola (page 72) and yogurt	Peanut butter and jelly on low-FODMAP bread and baby spinach salad with leftover Goddess Dressing (page 179)
T	Peanut butter and leftover Strawberry-Lemon Chia Seed Jam (page 183) on low-FODMAP toast	Leftover Banana–Chocolate Chip Oatmeal Bite (page 85)	Leftover Barbecue Pulled Pork (page 151) with a low-FODMAP bun and Classic Coleslaw with a Lime Twist (page 95)
F	Banana and Peanut Butter Oatmeal Bowl (page 79)	Leftover Roasted Red Pepper Hummus (page 163) and carrots	Leftover Sheet Pan Chicken and Vegetables (page 148) in a tortilla wrap
S	Quinoa-Berry Breakfast Bake (page 82)	Leftover Peanut Butter Power Balls (page 168)	Loaded Nachos (page 118)
S	Leftover Broccoli and Cheese Frittata (page 109) with low-FODMAP toast	Leftover Trail Mix (page 160)	Comforting Chicken Soup (page 92) with a low-FODMAP bun

SNACK	DINNER	NOTES
Leftover Peanut Butter Power Balls (page 168)	Spaghetti Bolognese (page 154) with Caesar Salad (page 98)	
Grapes and Cheddar cheese	Canadian Maple Salmon (page 131) and baby spinach salad with Goddess Dressing (page 179)	
Leftover Peanut Butter Power Balls (page 168)	Barbecue Pulled Pork (page 151) with a low-FODMAP bun and Classic Coleslaw with a Lime Twist (page 95)	
Leftover Roasted Red Pepper Hummus (page 163) and cucumber	Sheet Pan Chicken and Vegetables (page 148)	
Leftover Trail Mix (page 160)	Broccoli and Cheese Frittata (page 109) with Carrot-Ginger Soup (page 90)	
Orange	Turkey Burgers (page 149) with Sriracha Mayonnaise (page 182) on a low-FODMAP bun with Cajun-Spiced Root Vegetable Fries (page 103)	
Fresh Cut Salsa (page 177) and tortilla chips	Lentil Shepherd's Pie (page 119)	

Canned and bottled items

- Beans, black, 1 (16-ounce) can
- Lentils, 1 (15-ounce) can
- Mayonnaise, 1 (8-ounce) jar*
- Mustard, Dijon, smooth, 1 (8-ounce) jar
- Olives, black, 1 (6-ounce) can
- Soy sauce, 1 (10-ounce) bottle
- Sriracha, 1 (17-ounce) bottle
- Tabasco sauce, 1 (2-ounce) bottle (optional)
- Tomato paste, 1 (6-ounce) can
- Tomato sauce, 1 (15-ounce) can
- Worcestershire sauce, 1 (10-ounce) bottle

Dairy and eggs

- Butter (8 ounces)
- Cheese, Cheddar (8 ounces)
- Cheese, Parmesan, grated (¾ cup)
- Eggs, large (10)
- Milk, lactose-free or almond (½ gallon)
- Yogurt, plain, lactose-free (16 ounces)

Meat

- Bacon bits (½ cup) (optional)
- Beef, ground, lean (8 ounces)
- Chicken, boneless, skinless breasts or thighs (12 ounces)
- Chicken, drumsticks (2 or 3)
- Pork, tenderloin (1 pound)
- Salmon, 1 (6-ounce) fillet
- Turkey, ground (4 ounces)

Pantry items

- Anchovy paste
- Banana chips
- Bay leaves
- Bread*
- Buns, hamburger*
- Cereal, Crispix
- Chocolate chips
- Cinnamon, ground
- Chia seeds
- Cocoa powder
- Dried cranberries or raisins
- Ginger, ground
- Italian seasoning*
- Jam
- Maple syrup
- Mustard, dry
- Nutritional yeast
- Oats, rolled
- Oil, coconut
- Oil, olive, extra-virgin

- Oregano, dried

- Paprika, smoked

- Peanut butter

- Peanuts, salted

- Peppercorns, black

- Puffed rice

- Quinoa

- Rosemary, dried

- Salt

- Spaghetti,
  low-FODMAP*

- Sugar, brown
  (optional)

- Sugar, light brown

- Sugar, white

- Thyme, dried

- Tortilla chips*

- Vinegar, apple cider

- Vinegar, red-wine

- Vinegar, rice-wine

- Walnuts

Produce

- Bananas, unripe (2)

- Beans, green
  (10 ounces)

- Blueberries (6 ounces)

- Broccoli (1 head)

- Carrots, medium (10)

- Celery (1 bunch)

- Cilantro (1 bunch)

- Coleslaw mix
  (14 ounces)

- Cucumber (1)

- Fennel (1 small bulb)

- Garlic (1 head)

- Ginger, fresh
  (1 small knob)

- Grapes (6 ounces)

- Kale (1 bunch)

- Leek (1 bunch)

- Lemons (2)

- Lettuce, romaine
  (1 head)

- Limes (3)

- Mushrooms, oyster
  (4 ounces)

- Orange (1)

- Parsley (1 bunch)

- Parsnip, small (1)

- Pepper, red bell (1)

- Pepper, jalapeño (1)
  (optional)

- Potatoes, yellow or
  red, medium (6)

- Raspberries (1 pint)

- Scallions (3 bunches)

- Strawberries
  (2 pounds)

- Spinach, baby
  (6 ounces)

- Sweet potato, small (1)

- Tomatoes (7)

- Zucchini, small (1)

*Read the ingredient list,
and avoid products with
high-FODMAP ingredients.

Week Three

Have a look at your week three meal plan, and fill in your grocery list before your trip to the grocery store. Do you have any special events in your agenda? It can be tempting to take a low-FODMAP day off, but remember you have many low-FODMAP options, even while eating out. Look at the menu online before you go, and don't be shy about asking your server for modifications. Any good restaurant would be happy to oblige. For more excellent tips, see Audrey's blog post on dining out (http://www.ibsnutrition.com /dining-low-fodmap-diet/).

RATE YOUR SYMPTOMS

If your symptoms have resolved completely or you are enjoying mostly symptom-free days, you can start the Reintroduction Phase (page 66). If you aren't quite there yet, keep your chin up, keep going, and check in on your symptoms using a scale of 1 to 10 (1 is low, 10 is high) and the Bristol Stool Chart to record your bowel movements.

BLOATING	
GAS PRODUCTION	
ABDOMINAL PAIN OR DISCOMFORT	
BOWEL MOVEMENTS	

PREPARATION TIPS

Make Ahead

- Banana-Carrot Muffins (page 172)

- Tzatziki Dip (page 167)

- ½ recipe Pumpkin Spice Chia Pudding (page 81)

Freeze

- Banana-Carrot Muffins (defrost one at a time before eating)

- 2 chicken breasts

Plan Ahead

- Wednesday: Make ¾ cup (dry) rice for Wednesday and Thursday

PREPARATION NOTES

For the following recipes this week, you will make only a portion of the recipe as follows:

- ½ recipe Pumpkin Spice Chia Pudding (page 81)

- ½ recipe Italian Pork Patties (page 75)

- ½ recipe Savory or Sweet Crêpes (page 83)

- ½ recipe Chile-Lime DIY Tacos (page 153)

- ½ recipe Coconut Chicken Strips (page 142)

- ⅓ recipe Warm Roasted Vegetable Salad (page 104)

- ¼ recipe Fish in a Bag (page 139)

- ½ recipe Thai Peanut Stir-Fry (page 115)

- ½ recipe Sweet Potato Quinoa Cakes (page 97)

- ¼ recipe Cranberry-Quinoa Salad (page 100)

WEEK THREE MENU AT A GLANCE

	BREAKFAST	SNACK	LUNCH
M	Leftover Quinoa-Berry Breakfast Bake (page 82)	Leftover Peanut Butter Power Balls (page 168)	Leftover Comforting Chicken Soup (page 92)
T	Pumpkin Spice Chia Pudding (page 81)	Leftover Tzatziki Dip (page 167) and red bell pepper slices	Leftover Chile-Lime DIY Tacos (page 153) with Fresh Cut Salsa (page 177)
W	Raspberry Cheesecake Smoothie (page 77)	Leftover Pumpkin Spice Chia Pudding (page 81)	Leftover chopped up Coconut Chicken Strips (page 142) on spinach salad
T	Peanut butter on low-FODMAP toast with strawberries	Leftover Peanut Butter Power Balls (page 168)	Ham and cheese sandwich with leftover Warm Roasted Vegetable Salad (page 104)
F	Leftover Banana–Chocolate Chip Oatmeal Bite (page 85)	Banana-Carrot Muffin (page 172)	Leftover Thai Peanut Stir-Fry (page 115) with rice
S	Italian Pork Patties (page 75) with scrambled eggs	Leftover Sunshine Granola (page 72) and milk	Savory Smoked Salmon Crêpes (page 83)
S	Sweet Crêpes (page 83) with strawberries	Leftover Peanut Butter Power Balls (page 168)	Tofu BLT (page 116) with ½ cup red bell pepper slices

SNACK	DINNER	NOTES
Tzatziki Dip (page 167) with cucumbers	Chile-Lime DIY Tacos (page 153) with leftover Fresh Cut Salsa (page 177)	
Leftover Sunshine Granola (page 72)	Coconut Chicken Strips (page 142) with Warm Roasted Vegetable Salad (page 104)	
Leftover Tzatziki Dip (page 167) with carrots	Fish in a Bag (page 139) with rice	
Leftover Banana–Chocolate Chip Oatmeal Bite (page 85)	Thai Peanut Stir-Fry (page 115) with rice	
Leftover Pumpkin Spice Chia Pudding (page 81)	Sweet Potato Quinoa Cakes (page 97) with Chive-Rubbed Chicken (page 143)	
Flourless Peanut Butter– Banana Cookies (page 162)	Lentil-Squash Stew (page 121)	
Leftover Banana-Carrot Muffin (page 172)	Cranberry-Quinoa Salad (page 100) with leftover Chive-Rubbed Chicken (page 143)	

SHOPPING LIST

Canned and bottled items

- Beans, black,
  1 (16-ounce) can

- Coconut milk, full-fat,
  2 (13½-ounce) cans

- Juice, cranberry,
  100-percent*
  (4 ounces)

- Lentils,
  2 (15-ounce) cans

- Mayonnaise,
  1 (8-ounce) jar*

- Mustard, Dijon,
  smooth,
  1 (8-ounce) jar

- Pumpkin purée,
  1 (15-ounce) can

- Soy sauce,
  1 (10-ounce) bottle

- Tomatoes, diced,
  1 (14½-ounce) can

- Tomato paste,
  1 (6-ounce) can

Dairy and eggs

- Butter (8 ounces)

- Cheese, Cheddar
  (3 ounces)

- Cheese, goat,
  crumbled (¼ cup)

- Cream cheese
  (8 ounces)

- Eggs, large (11)

- Mayonnaise

- Milk, lactose-free or
  almond (½ gallon)

- Sour cream,
  lactose-free (¼ cup)

- Yogurt, plain, Greek
  lactose-free
  (16 ounces)

Frozen foods

- Raspberries
  (8 ounces)

Meat

- Beef, ground, lean
  (4 ounces)

- Chicken, boneless,
  skinless breasts
  (1½ pounds)

- Ham, cooked, sliced (3 ounces)

- Pork, ground, extra lean (8 ounces)

- Salmon, smoked (5 ounces)

- Tilapia (4 ounces)

Pantry items

- Almond butter

- Almond meal

- Ancho chile powder*

- Baking soda

- Basil, dried

- Bay leaves

- Bread*

- Bread crumbs

- Cayenne

- Chia seeds

- Chives, dried

- Chocolate chips

- Cinnamon, ground

- Cloves, ground

- Coconut, dried, shredded, unsweetened

- Cranberries, dried

- Cumin, ground

- Dill, dried

- Flour blend, low-FODMAP*

- Flour, oat

- Flour, sweet or glutinous rice

- Ginger, ground

- Italian seasoning*

- Maple syrup

- Nonstick cooking spray

- Nutmeg, ground

- Oats, rolled

- Oil, coconut

- Oil, olive, extra-virgin

- Oil, sesame

- Oregano, dried

- Paprika

- Peanut butter

- Peppercorns, black

- Pumpkin seeds

- Quinoa

- Rice, white, long-grain

- Salt

- Sugar, brown

- Sugar, white

- Thyme, dried

- Tortillas, corn
  (4 small or 2 large)

- Turmeric, ground

- Vanilla extract

- Vinegar, balsamic

- Vinegar, red-wine

- Walnuts

Produce

- Bananas (3)

- Basil, fresh (1 bunch)

- Basil, Thai, fresh
  (1 bunch)

- Beans, green
  (10 ounces)

- Bell peppers, red (2)

- Broccoli (1 head)

- Carrots, medium (7)

- Cilantro (1 bunch)

- Cucumbers (2)

- Dill (1 bunch)

- Fennel (1)

- Ginger, fresh
  (1 small knob)

- Kale (1 bunch)

- Leek (1)

- Lemon (1)

- Lettuce, romaine
  (1 head)

- Limes (2)

- Mushrooms, oyster
  (4 ounces)

- Parsley (1 bunch)

- Potato, yellow or red,
  small (1)

- Scallions (2 bunches)

- Spinach, baby,
  1 (6-ounce) bag

- Squash, kabocha
  (1¾ pounds)

- Strawberries
  (1 pound)

- Sweet potato, small (1)

- Tomatoes (5)

- Tomatoes, cherry
  (1 pint)

- Zucchini, small (1)

Other

- Tofu, extra-firm,
  1 (14-ounce)
  package

*Read the ingredient list,
and avoid products with
high-FODMAP ingredients.

Week Four

Ironically, by week four, many people want to stay on this diet forever because they feel so much better. Monash recommends a two- to six-week trial of the diet and then moving on to the Reintroduction Phase. Check out your yummy meal plan for week four to finish on a strong note.

RATE YOUR SYMPTOMS

If your symptoms have completely resolved and you are enjoying mostly symptom-free days, you can start the Reintroduction Phase (page 66). If you still have some improvements to make, check in on your symptoms using a scale of 1 to 10 (1 is low, 10 is high) and the Bristol Stool Chart to record your bowel movements.

BLOATING	
GAS PRODUCTION	
ABDOMINAL PAIN OR DISCOMFORT	
BOWEL MOVEMENTS	

Make Ahead

- Olive Lover's Hummus (page 164)

- No-Bake Bars (page 161)

- Caesar Vinaigrette (page 188)

- Maple–Balsamic Vinegar Dressing (page 181)

Plan Ahead

- Sunday: Chop carrots, potatoes, and beef for Slow Cooker Beef Stew (page 157) to have it ready for Monday morning.

- The following Sunday (day 28): Buy the pork tenderloin so it is fresh. Marinate the pork around lunchtime so it's ready to grill by dinnertime.

PREPARATION NOTES

For the following recipes this week, you will make portions of the recipe as follows:

- Double recipe Chive-Rubbed Chicken (page 143)

- ¼ recipe Shrimp Fettuccine (page 137)

- ½ recipe Caesar Salad (page 98)

- ½ recipe Roasted Red Pepper Hippy Bowl (page 123)

- ½ recipe Ginger-Lime Salmon Burgers (page 135)

- ½ recipe Classic Coleslaw with a Lime Twist (page 95)

- ½ recipe Crispy Tofu (page 113)

- ⅓ recipe Crispy Parmesan Baby Potatoes (page 101)

- ¼ recipe Caprese Salad (page 93)

WEEK FOUR MENU AT A GLANCE

	BREAKFAST	SNACK	LUNCH
M	2 leftover "Rise and Shine" Egg Muffins (page 74)	Leftover Banana–Chocolate Chip Oatmeal Bite (page 85)	Leftover Lentil-Squash Stew (page 121)
T	Leftover Italian Pork Patties (page 75) with eggs	No-Bake Bars (page 161)	Leftover Slow Cooker Beef Stew (page 157)
W	Banana and Peanut Butter Oatmeal Bowl (page 79)	Olive Lover's Hummus (page 164) and rice crackers	Leftover Chive-Rubbed Chicken (page 143) sandwich and carrots
T	2 leftover Banana–Chocolate Chip Oatmeal Bites (page 85)	1 leftover "Rise and Shine" Egg Muffin (page 74) and an orange	Leftover Caesar Salad (page 98) with Chive-Rubbed Chicken (page 143)
F	Oatmeal Cookie Smoothie (page 78)	An orange and leftover No-Bake Bars (page 161)	Leftover Olive Lover's Hummus (page 164) with carrots, cheese, and crackers
S	Banana Egg Pancakes (page 87)	Cheese and an orange	Grilled cheese and leftover Classic Coleslaw with a Lime Twist (page 95)
S	Baked French Toast (page 73) with 1 cup strawberries	Leftover No-Bake Bars (page 161)	Leftover Crispy Tofu (page 113) in a wrap with spinach

SNACK	DINNER	NOTES
Leftover Cranberry-Quinoa Salad (page 100)	Slow Cooker Beef Stew (page 157)	
1 leftover "Rise and Shine" Egg Muffin (page 74)	Feta, Tomato, and Spinach Rice (page 99) with Chive-Rubbed Chicken (page 143)	
Leftover No-Bake Bars (page 161)	Shrimp Fettuccine (page 137) with Caesar Salad (page 98)	
Leftover Olive Lover's Hummus (page 164) and red bell pepper slices	Roasted Red Pepper Hippy Bowl (page 123) with steamed carrots	
Leftover Trail Mix (page 160)	Ginger-Lime Salmon Burger (page 135) with Classic Coleslaw with a Lime Twist (page 95)	
Chocolate-Walnut Brownies (page 169)	Crispy Tofu (page 113), Crispy Parmesan Baby Potatoes (page 101), and green salad with Maple–Balsamic Vinegar Dressing (page 181)	
Oatmeal Cookie Smoothie (page 78)	Pork Tenderloin Medallions (page 150) with Caprese Salad (page 93) and leftover Crispy Parmesan Baby Potatoes (page 101)	

Canned and bottled items

- Chickpeas,
  1 (15½-ounce) can

- Cooking wine, white,
  1 (16-ounce) bottle

- Lentils,
  1 (15-ounce) can

- Mayonnaise,
  1 (8-ounce) jar*

- Mustard, Dijon,
  smooth,
  1 (8-ounce) jar

- Olives, Kalamata,
  pitted (½ cup)

- Roasted red peppers,
  1 (12-ounce) jar

- Salmon, boneless,
  skinless,
  1 (6-ounce) can

- Soy sauce,
  1 (10-ounce) bottle

- Tabasco sauce,
  1 (2-ounce) bottle

- Tomato juice
  (32 ounces)

Dairy and eggs

- Butter (8 ounces)

- Cheese, bocconcini
  (1 ounce)

- Cheese, Cheddar
  (5 ounces)

- Cheese, feta
  (8 ounces)

- Cheese, Parmesan,
  grated (½ cup)

- Eggs (11)

- Half-and-half, lactose-
  free (2 ounces)

- Milk, lactose-free or
  almond (½ gallon)

Meat

- Bacon bits (¼ cup)
  (optional)

- Beef, for stew
  (1 pound)

- Chicken, boneless,
  skinless breasts,
  2 (8-ounce) fillets

- Pork, tenderloin
  (1 pound)

- Shrimp, peeled and
  deveined (4 ounces)

Pantry items

- Almond butter

- Almond flour

- Anchovy paste

- Baking powder

- Basil, dried

- Bay leaves

- Bread crumbs,
  gluten-free

- Brown rice syrup

- Buns, hamburger*

- Cereal, puffed rice

- Chives, dried

- Chocolate chips,
  semisweet

- Cinnamon, ground

- Cocoa powder

- Cornstarch

- Crackers, rice*

- Cranberries, dried

- Cumin, ground

- Fettuccine,
  low-FODMAP*

- Flour, almond

- Flour blend,
  low-FODMAP*

- Maple syrup

- Nonstick
  cooking spray

- Nutmeg, ground
  (optional)

- Oats, rolled

- Oil, olive, extra-virgin

- Oil, sesame

- Paprika

- Peanut butter

- Peppercorns, black

- Quinoa

- Rice, basmati

- Salt

- Sugar, brown

- Sugar, white

- Tortillas, corn

- Vanilla extract

- Vinegar, balsamic

- Vinegar, red-wine

- Walnuts

Produce

- Bananas, unripe (6)

- Basil (1 bunch)

- Carrots (11)

- Coleslaw mix
  (14 ounces)

- Fennel (1)

- Garlic (1 head)

- Ginger, fresh
  (1 small knob)

- Kale (1 bunch)

- Leek (1)

- Lemon (1)

- Lettuce, romaine
  (1 head)

- Lime (1)

- Mushrooms, oyster
  (4 ounces)

- Oranges (5)

- Parsley (1 bunch)

- Pepper, red bell (1)

- Potatoes, yellow or
  red, medium (2)

- Potatoes, baby
  (8 ounces)

- Scallions (1 bunch)

- Spinach, baby
  (6 ounces)

- Tomato (4)

- Zucchini (1 small)

Other

- Tofu, extra-firm,
  1 (14-ounce) package

*Read the ingredient list,
and avoid products with
high-FODMAP ingredients.

Beyond the Four Weeks— Reintroduction and FODMAP Personalization

You have worked hard to get here. We're proud of you! Now, put on your scientist hat because this is where you systematically test selected high-FODMAP foods to find out which types and amounts of FODMAPs trigger symptoms. We find this to be the most interesting part, but it can feel like a marathon. You will likely have a plethora of questions, which is why Monash recommends enlisting the help of a Monash FODMAP-trained dietitian.

FODMAP REINTRODUCTION

Is the thought of eating high-FODMAP foods again terrifying? You're not alone in that feeling, but trust us, completing this next phase is worth it. You may find that you can happily eat many high-FODMAP foods again. Wouldn't that be great? You may discover that some need to be limited, and a select few may be your own version of evil (like garlic for Joanna Baker). Either way, knowledge is power.

Here are the key points:

- Continue to eat a low-FODMAP diet. Try eating the 28-day meal plan again for the next four weeks.

- Choose a food that contains only one high-FODMAP group. Examples of foods and the amounts are found in the diary section of the Monash app. You can test the foods in any order.

- Start with the small serving on day one, medium on day two, and large on day three. You can skip days in between if you like.

- Stop if significant symptoms return.

- Record the food, the amounts, and any symptoms (if you had them).

- Have a washout period of about two days with no symptoms before you start the next test.

- If you have no symptoms, you must still avoid that FODMAP group until you have finished all of the testing.

- In a few weeks, you can retest foods that triggered symptoms, as your tolerance for FODMAPs can change over time.

FODMAP PERSONALIZATION

Once you are done with FODMAP reintroduction, it's time to move on to "personalization." It may feel like a 180-degree change in thinking because your new goal is to enjoy as much variety and FODMAPs as possible without symptoms. Audrey likes to call this "toeing the line."

Make a list of the FODMAP groups that triggered symptoms, including the serving size when the symptoms started. If you had symptoms with the smallest serving size, avoid this group completely for now. If your symptoms started after the medium or large servings, you can enjoy a small amount of these foods. Make a list of the FODMAP groups that you tested in the largest serving size without experiencing any symptoms. You can slowly begin eating these foods again.

In the long run, you can retest high-FODMAP foods to see if your body is better able to digest them over time.

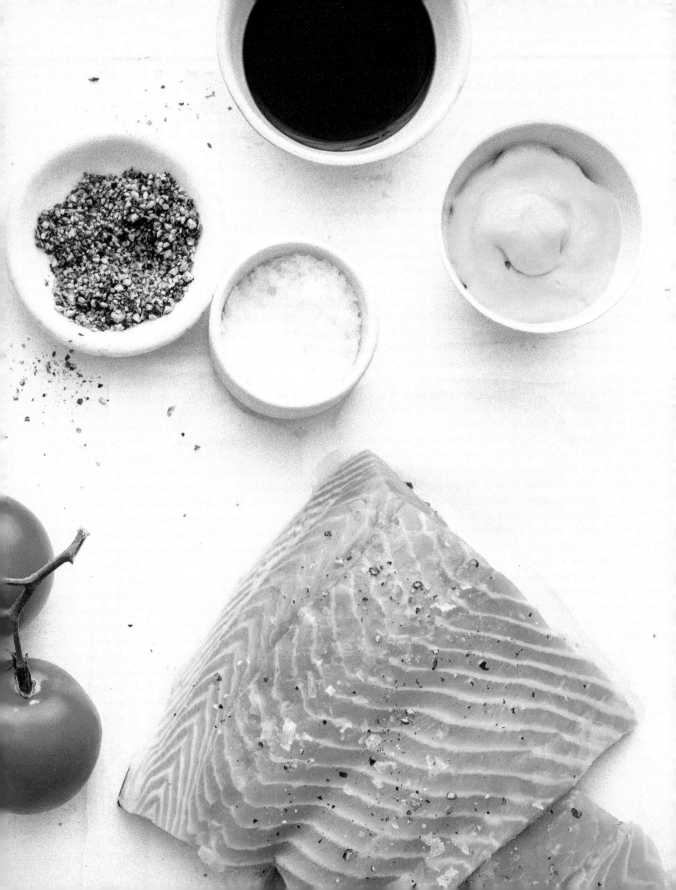

PART TWO

LOW-FODMAP RECIPES

Our recipes are very simple and use everyday ingredients. You'll probably recognize some as being like your home-cooked favorites, but with low-FODMAP ingredients. Each recipe is clearly laid out with several labels and tips.

For recipes without any animal products or without seafood and meat, you'll see Vegan and Vegetarian labels, respectively. The Gluten-Free label means that the recipes do not include any gluten-containing grains (i.e., wheat, barley, or rye). A special note for our gluten-free readers: Always check ingredient packaging for gluten-free labeling in order to ensure foods, especially oats, were processed in a completely gluten-free facility.

Recipes with few ingredients, and/or are done in 30 minutes or less, are noted with 5 Ingredients or Less and 30 Minutes or Less labels, respectively, and as applicable. Recipes that work well when made in advance have a Make Ahead label, and recipes that have easy cleanup because they are made all in one pot are labeled as One Pot dishes.

Always be mindful of serving size, as larger portions can sometimes make the meal high-FODMAP.

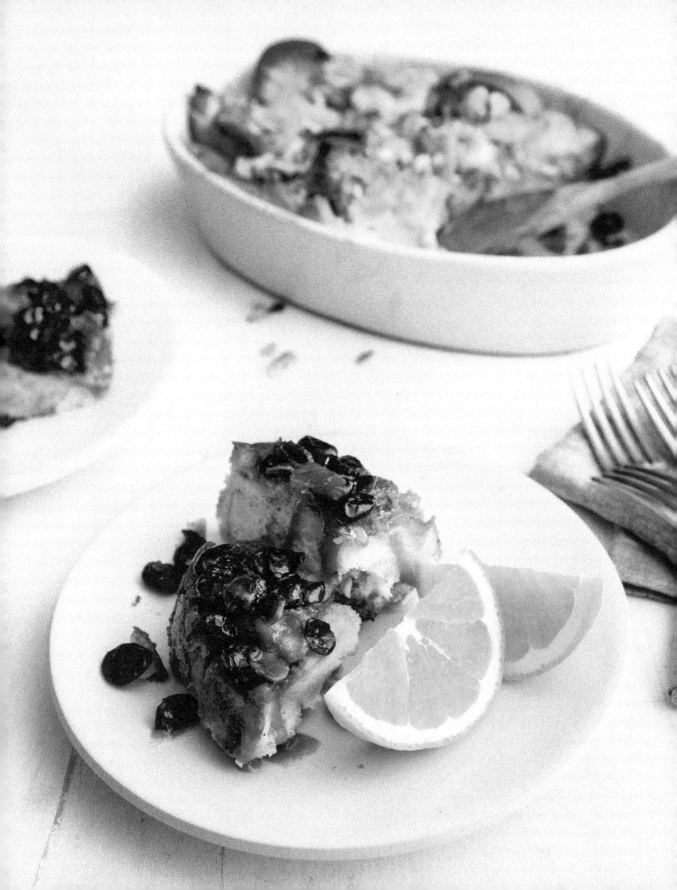

CHAPTER FOUR

Breakfast and Smoothies

Baked French Toast, page 73

Sunshine Granola

VEGAN • MAKE AHEAD • ONE POT

SERVES 11 [½ CUP = 1 SERVING] / PREP TIME: 10 MINUTES / COOK TIME: 40 MINUTES

In less than 10 minutes, your kitchen will smell like sweet orange and cinnamon with this lovely granola in your oven. Granola is quick to assemble and stores well in an airtight container. Store-bought granola is typically riddled with high-FODMAP ingredients, but you won't miss it after trying this scrumptious recipe. Enjoy it with lactose-free yogurt and a dollop of the Strawberry-Lemon Chia Seed Jam (page 183).

4 cups rolled oats

1½ cups coarsely chopped walnuts

1 teaspoon ground cinnamon

½ cup coconut oil, melted

½ cup maple syrup

Grated zest of 1 orange

1. Preheat the oven to 350°F. Line a large sheet pan with parchment paper.
2. In a large mixing bowl, combine the oats, walnuts, and cinnamon.
3. In a small bowl, mix together the oil, maple syrup, and orange zest.
4. Add the wet ingredients to the oats, and mix until everything is well coated.
5. Spread the granola evenly on the prepared sheet pan.
6. Transfer the sheet pan to the oven, and bake, rotating halfway through, for 40 minutes, or until the oats are golden brown. Remove from the oven, and let cool. Store in an airtight container for up to 1 month.

VARIATION TIP: For a richer flavor, you can use melted butter instead of coconut oil.

FODMAP TIP: A low-FODMAP serving is ½ cup. If you use quick oats, the low-FODMAP serving size is ¼ cup.

Per Serving (½ cup): Calories: 347; Total Fat: 22g; Saturated Fat: 10g; Cholesterol: 0mg; Sodium: 3mg; Carbohydrates: 33g; Fiber: 5g; Protein: 6g

Baked French Toast

VEGETARIAN • MAKE AHEAD • ONE POT

SERVES 4 / PREP TIME: 15 MINUTES / COOK TIME: 45 MINUTES

This dish is a weekend staple in Audrey's house. Her husband, Dave, prepares it in the evening and keeps it covered in the refrigerator overnight so that it is ready to go in the oven first thing in the morning. It is the perfect dish for a weekend brunch with friends or if you need to hit the ground running with a nutritious meal in your belly. Serve it with the Italian Pork Patties (page 75) for a perfect combination of salty and sweet.

4 tablespoons (½ stick) butter, melted

¼ cup dried cranberries

⅓ cup lightly packed brown sugar

¼ cup chopped walnuts

8 slices low-FODMAP bread

4 large eggs, beaten

½ cup lactose-free milk or almond milk

1 teaspoon vanilla extract

1 teaspoon ground cinnamon

Maple syrup, for serving (optional)

1. Preheat the oven to 350°F.

2. In a small pot, warm the butter, cranberries, and sugar over medium-low heat for 5 minutes, or until the butter has melted and the cranberries have softened. Pour into an 8-inch square baking dish, and spread it evenly across the bottom.

3. Top with the walnuts.

4. Roughly tear each slice of bread into 4 or 5 pieces, and fill the baking dish.

5. In a medium bowl, whisk together the eggs, milk, vanilla, and cinnamon. Pour evenly over the bread.

6. Gently press down on the bread to encourage it to soak up the egg mixture.

7. Transfer the baking dish to the oven, and bake for 40 minutes, or until the top is brown and the middle has cooked through. Remove from the oven.

8. Divide the French toast among 4 plates. Top with the cranberries from the bottom of the baking dish. Serve with maple syrup (if using).

COOKING TIP: You can prepare this dish the night before and store it covered in the refrigerator so that it is ready to go in the oven in the morning.

Per Serving: Calories: 477; Total Fat: 24g; Saturated Fat: 10g; Cholesterol: 217mg; Sodium: 341mg; Carbohydrates: 52g; Fiber: 5g; Protein: 15g

"Rise and Shine" Egg Muffins

VEGETARIAN · GLUTEN-FREE · 30 MINUTES OR LESS · MAKE AHEAD · ONE POT

SERVES 6 / PREP TIME: 10 MINUTES / COOK TIME: 20 MINUTES

We think that every day should start with a great source of protein like these little Mediterranean-inspired egg cups. Not only are they delicious and easy to prepare, but also they are very versatile. You can have them for breakfast or lunch or as a high-protein post-workout snack. Audrey finds that cooking spray is the best way to prevent them from sticking.

Nonstick cooking spray, for greasing

10 large eggs

1 cup chopped spinach

1 cup crumbled feta cheese

½ cup finely chopped red bell pepper

¼ cup chopped scallions, green

**   parts only**

¼ teaspoon salt

Freshly ground black pepper

1. Preheat the oven to 350°F. Grease a 12-cup muffin tin.
2. In a large mixing bowl, whisk together the eggs.
3. Add the spinach, cheese, bell pepper, scallions, and salt. Season with pepper.
4. Divide the egg mixture among the prepared muffin tin cups.
5. Transfer the muffin tin to the oven, and bake for 20 minutes, or until the tops of the muffins have lightly browned. Remove from the oven.
6. Use a butter knife to loosen the muffins, remove them from the tin, and let cool.

VARIATION TIP: You can use any type of cheese like mozzarella, Cheddar, or smoked Cheddar. You can swap the red pepper for an equal portion of green pepper, broccoli, tomato, or zucchini.

FODMAP TIP: A low-FODMAP serving is 2 muffins.

COOKING TIP: Make a double recipe, and store the muffins in the freezer. Defrost when you are ready to eat.

Per Serving: Calories: 191; Total Fat: 14g; Saturated Fat: 6g; Cholesterol: 332mg; Sodium: 412mg; Carbohydrates: 3g; Fiber: 0g; Protein: 14g

Italian Pork Patties

GLUTEN-FREE • 5 INGREDIENTS OR LESS •
30 MINUTES OR LESS • MAKE AHEAD • ONE POT

SERVES 4 / PREP TIME: 5 MINUTES / COOK TIME: 15 MINUTES

Instead of spending your time searching for low-FODMAP packaged sausages, you'll be pleasantly surprised by how quick and delicious these patties are. Serve them with your favorite eggs, low-FODMAP toast, and a piece of low-FODMAP fruit for a perfect weekend brunch or leisurely breakfast. These patties are totally unprocessed, with less salt, more nutrition, and better flavor than your conventional sausages.

1 pound extra-lean ground pork

2 teaspoons Italian seasoning

¾ teaspoon salt

1. In a medium bowl, combine the pork, Italian seasoning, and salt, and mix well.
2. Shape ¼-cup portions of the mixture into 8 (1-inch-thick) patties.
3. Heat a large skillet over medium-high heat until hot.
4. Add the patties, and cook, flipping once, for 7 minutes per side, or until browned and cooked through.

COOKING TIP: You can double the recipe and store extras in the freezer. Defrost them in the refrigerator when you are ready to eat them.

VARIATION TIP: Use ground chicken or turkey instead of pork.

Per Serving: Calories: 180; Total Fat: 4g; Saturated Fat: 2g; Cholesterol: 90mg; Sodium: 548mg; Carbohydrates: 0g; Fiber: 0g; Protein: 35g

Peanut Butter and Chocolate Smoothie

**VEGETARIAN • GLUTEN-FREE • 5 INGREDIENTS OR LESS •
30 MINUTES OR LESS • ONE POT**

SERVES 1 / PREP TIME: 5 MINUTES

In Audrey's household, smoothies are so popular that her family has literally worn out multiple blenders. This smoothie is why you should keep unripe bananas in your freezer at all times. It is a perfect high-protein post-workout snack and a total crowd pleaser when you have a kitchen full of hungry kids.

1 unripe banana, frozen

**½ cup lactose-free milk, plus more
   as needed**

1 tablespoon peanut butter

1 teaspoon cocoa powder

In a blender, combine the banana, milk, peanut butter, and cocoa. Blend until smooth. If it is too thick, add more milk.

SUBSTITUTION TIP: For a vegan variation, use almond milk.

COOKING TIP: Peel and freeze bananas in a freezer bag. Label them with a Sharpie marker as either "unripe" or "ripe."

VARIATION TIP: Add frozen baby spinach or kale to pump up the nutrition.

FODMAP TIP: If you use a ripe banana instead of unripe, use only one-third of the banana, as the FODMAP content of bananas increases as they ripen.

Per Serving: Calories: 283; Total Fat: 12g; Saturated Fat: 2g; Cholesterol: 0mg; Sodium: 185mg; Carbohydrates: 44g; Fiber: 6g; Protein: 7g

Raspberry Cheesecake Smoothie

VEGETARIAN • GLUTEN-FREE • 30 MINUTES OR LESS • ONE POT

SERVES 1 / PREP TIME: 5 MINUTES

This recipe earned its name for obvious reasons. It is like eating raspberry cheesecake ice cream. It is thick, rich, and luxurious. You may feel like you are cheating, but you're not. Our rule of thumb for smoothies is that they must be packed full of nutrition so that they are like a mini meal. This one is high in protein and fiber, which means that it makes for a healthy breakfast or snack.

½ cup frozen raspberries

½ cup plain Greek lactose-free yogurt

½ cup lactose-free milk

1 tablespoon cream cheese

1 tablespoon chia seeds

1 tablespoon maple syrup

4 ice cubes

In a blender, combine the raspberries, yogurt, milk, cream cheese, chia seeds, maple syrup, and ice. Blend until smooth. If it is too thick, add more milk.

SUBSTITUTION TIP: For a vegan smoothie, use plain coconut yogurt, almond milk, and vegan cream cheese. Watch for high-FODMAP ingredients like inulin or chicory root in the coconut yogurt and vegan cream cheese.

INGREDIENT TIP: For a lighter smoothie, use nonfat Greek yogurt and lactose-free skim milk, and omit the cream cheese.

FODMAP TIP: Cream cheese is naturally low in lactose. One tablespoon contains 1 gram of lactose, which is a low-FODMAP serving.

Per Serving: Calories: 278; Total Fat: 10g; Saturated Fat: 3g; Cholesterol: 13mg; Sodium: 148mg; Carbohydrates: 35g; Fiber: 10g; Protein: 15g

Oatmeal Cookie Smoothie

VEGETARIAN • 30 MINUTES OR LESS • ONE POT

SERVES 1 / PREP TIME: 5 MINUTES

This is a cool and creamy smoothie with a flavor reminiscent of a fresh batch of oatmeal cookies. Plus, unlike cookies, it's packed with nutrition. If you want to make this smoothie sweeter, you can add a teaspoon of maple syrup or sugar. We recommend making the smoothie without any added sugar first and tasting it. We think it's sweet and flavorful enough to not need added sugar.

1 unripe banana, sliced and frozen

¾ cup lactose-free milk or almond milk

¼ cup ice cubes

2 tablespoons rolled oats

1 tablespoon almond butter

½ teaspoon ground cinnamon

⅛ teaspoon vanilla extract

Pinch ground nutmeg (optional)

In a blender, combine the banana, milk, ice, oats, almond butter, cinnamon, vanilla, and nutmeg (if using). Blend until smooth. If it is too thick, add more milk.

VARIATION TIP: Throw in some frozen baby spinach or kale to up the nutrition. Add peanut butter instead of almond butter.

Per Serving: Calories: 309; Total Fat: 15g; Saturated Fat: 1g; Cholesterol: 0mg; Sodium: 273mg; Carbohydrates: 40g; Fiber: 8g; Protein: 8g

Banana and Peanut Butter Oatmeal Bowl

VEGETARIAN · 5 INGREDIENTS OR LESS ·
30 MINUTES OR LESS · MAKE AHEAD · ONE POT

SERVES 1 / PREP TIME: 1 MINUTE / COOK TIME: 10 MINUTES

Our all-time favorite oatmeal is this banana peanut butter bowl. When we started writing this book, we both knew this one had to be included. Oatmeal bowls are a quick and balanced breakfast, as oats are a whole grain and high in fiber. With the added banana and peanut butter, you will have a deliciously healthy breakfast.

½ **cup rolled oats**

¼ **teaspoon ground cinnamon**

1 **tablespoon peanut butter**

½ **medium unripe banana, sliced**

1 **teaspoon brown sugar (optional)**

2 **tablespoons lactose-free milk**

  (optional)

1. In a small pot, prepare the oats according to the package instructions. Scoop into a bowl.

2. Stir the cinnamon into the oats.

3. Swirl in the peanut butter.

4. Top with the banana slices, and sprinkle the sugar (if using) on top.

5. Pour in the milk (if using).

VARIATION TIP: Use lactose-free milk or almond milk instead of water to cook the oats for added nutrition.

FODMAP TIP: Quick or instant oats cook much faster than large flake oats, but quick oats are higher in FODMAPs than whole oats. If you would like to use quick oats, reduce the portion to ¼ cup of oats.

Per Serving: Calories: 298; Total Fat: 11g; Saturated Fat: 2g; Cholesterol: 0mg; Sodium: 76mg; Carbohydrates: 44g; Fiber: 7g; Protein: 10g

Vanilla-Maple Overnight Oats

VEGETARIAN · 5 INGREDIENTS OR LESS · MAKE AHEAD · ONE POT

SERVES 1 / PREP TIME: 5 MINUTES, PLUS OVERNIGHT TO SOAK

It takes only two minutes in the evening to combine all of the ingredients so you will have a complete breakfast to grab and go the next day. Because overnight oats don't need to be cooked, you can pack this recipe in a Mason jar and throw it in your bag to eat when you get to work. There are three key components to overnight oats: rolled oats, milk, and chia seeds. The chia seeds soak up extra liquid and greatly improve the texture, plus they add protein and soluble fiber.

⅔ cup lactose-free milk or almond milk

⅓ cup rolled oats

1 tablespoon chia seeds

1 teaspoon maple syrup

¼ teaspoon vanilla extract

1. In a small bowl, mix together the milk, oats, chia seeds, maple syrup, and vanilla. If you plan to take it with you in the morning, use a Mason jar or sealed container. Cover, and place in the refrigerator overnight.

2. In the morning, stir and add your desired toppings (see the Variation Tip). It can be served cold or warmed up in the microwave.

VARIATION TIP: There are wonderful combinations of toppings that pair nicely with this oatmeal such as pineapple and shredded coconut, strawberry and orange, or walnuts and half an unripe banana.

FODMAP TIP: Chia seeds and rolled oats can become high-FODMAP with a larger serving size.

Per Serving: Calories: 295; Total Fat: 11g; Saturated Fat: 1g; Cholesterol: 0mg; Sodium: 243mg; Carbohydrates: 39g; Fiber: 11g; Protein: 9g

Pumpkin Spice Chia Pudding

VEGETARIAN • GLUTEN-FREE • MAKE AHEAD • ONE POT

SERVES 6 / PREP TIME: 5 MINUTES, PLUS 2 HOURS TO THICKEN

This recipe is perfect for those who don't have a lot of time for breakfast. Simply mix all the ingredients together in a bowl, and let it thicken overnight in the refrigerator. The texture is like tapioca pudding. Lauren will make a big bowl full of pudding at the start of the week and eat it over the next five days. Enjoy it topped with chopped walnuts or unripe banana slices. Drink plenty of water when eating foods with a lot of fiber like chia seeds.

2½ cups lactose-free milk or almond milk

1½ cups canned pumpkin purée

½ cup chia seeds

¼ cup maple syrup or brown sugar

2 teaspoons ground cinnamon

1 teaspoon ground ginger

¼ teaspoon ground cloves

¼ teaspoon ground nutmeg

1. In a medium bowl, mix together the milk, pumpkin, chia seeds, maple syrup, cinnamon, ginger, cloves, and nutmeg. Let it sit for 5 minutes, then give it another stir. Cover, and let the pudding thicken in the refrigerator for at least 2 hours or overnight.

2. Taste the pudding, and add more spices as desired. Keep in the refrigerator for up to 5 days.

VARIATION TIP: Top the pudding with a small sprinkle of cinnamon, chopped walnuts, or banana slices.

FODMAP TIP: A low-FODMAP serving is one-sixth of the recipe or ¾ cup pudding.

Per Serving: Calories: 186; Total Fat: 9g; Saturated Fat: 1g; Cholesterol: 0mg; Sodium: 158mg; Carbohydrates: 24g; Fiber: 10g; Protein: 5g

Quinoa-Berry Breakfast Bake

VEGETARIAN · GLUTEN-FREE · MAKE AHEAD · ONE POT

SERVES 8 / PREP TIME: 5 MINUTES / COOK TIME: 1 HOUR

Try out something new for breakfast. The protein and fiber in this casserole will keep you full until lunchtime. Take an hour to bake this on the weekend, and continue to enjoy it over the next five days, or freeze it and enjoy it another week.

1 teaspoon butter

1½ cups quinoa

1½ cups chopped strawberries

1 cup blueberries

½ cup raspberries

¼ cup chopped walnuts (optional)

3 large eggs

3 cups lactose-free milk or almond milk

¼ cup brown sugar

1 tablespoon ground cinnamon

1 teaspoon ground ginger

1. Preheat the oven to 375°F. Grease a glass 9-by-13-inch baking dish.

2. Pour the quinoa into the baking dish, and lightly shake to distribute evenly.

3. Sprinkle the strawberries, blueberries, raspberries, and walnuts (if using) over the quinoa.

4. In a large bowl, whisk together the eggs. Stir in the milk, sugar, cinnamon, and ginger. Gently pour over the quinoa mixture.

5. Transfer the baking dish to the oven, and bake for 1 hour, or until the quinoa has absorbed all of the liquid. Slice into 8 pieces. Extra servings can be kept in the refrigerator for up to 5 days or in the freezer for months.

COOKING TIP: Double the recipe, and store it in individual portions in the freezer. It will keep in the freezer for a few months.

Per Serving: Calories: 223; Total Fat: 7g; Saturated Fat: 1g; Cholesterol: 71mg; Sodium: 168mg; Carbohydrates: 32g; Fiber: 5g; Protein: 8g

Savory or Sweet Crêpes

GLUTEN-FREE · ONE POT

SERVES 4 / PREP TIME: 5 MINUTES / COOK TIME: 30 MINUTES

Lauren's family affectionately refers to this recipe as "Swedish Pancakes," as the recipe is from her Swedish grandmother. Lauren worked on this recipe for weeks to make a low-FODMAP version that was as good as the original. It contains glutinous rice flour, which is well worth a trip to an Asian grocery store or bulk food store to find.

3 large eggs

1½ cups lactose-free 2-percent milk

¾ cup glutinous or sweet rice flour

1 tablespoon white sugar

1 teaspoon salt

2 tablespoons butter, divided

FOR THE SAVORY VERSION

10 ounces smoked salmon

½ cup crumbled goat cheese

¼ cup chopped fresh dill or 1 tablespoon dried dill

FOR THE SWEET VERSION

2 cups chopped strawberries

¼ cup maple syrup

1. To make the batter, in a large bowl, whisk the eggs well, then whisk in the milk, flour, sugar, and salt.

2. Heat a large skillet over medium-low heat. Melt and spread 1 teaspoon of butter in the pan.

3. Whisk the batter well until there are plenty of bubbles and no flour settled on the bottom. Pour ¼ cup into the middle of the pan. Gently tilt in a full circle so the batter spreads to cover the whole pan. Cook for 2 to 3 minutes, or until the bubbles in the batter have popped and the bottom has browned.

4. Flip the crêpe, and cook for 1 to 2 minutes, or until browned on the other side. Transfer to a large plate. Cover with another inverted plate to keep warm.

> CONTINUED ON NEXT PAGE

5. Before cooking another crêpe, melt and spread ½ teaspoon of butter in the pan and whisk the batter again until bubbles form. Repeat this step every time before pouring the batter into the pan. Continue making crêpes until all the butter and batter are used up.

6. Divide your toppings evenly among the crêpes, and serve.

VARIATION TIP: You can use a low-FODMAP flour blend instead of glutinous rice flour, but the texture may not be as good.

COOKING TIP: If possible, prepare the batter the night before. Cover and place in the refrigerator overnight.

SAVORY VERSION
Per Serving: Calories: 400; Total Fat: 18g; Saturated Fat: 9g; Cholesterol: 191mg; Sodium: 2182mg; Carbohydrates: 35g; Fiber: 1g; Protein: 26g

SWEET VERSION
Per Serving: Calories: 344; Total Fat: 12g; Saturated Fat: 6g; Cholesterol: 162mg; Sodium: 720mg; Carbohydrates: 52g; Fiber: 2g; Protein: 10g

Banana–Chocolate Chip Oatmeal Bites

VEGETARIAN · 30 MINUTES OR LESS · MAKE AHEAD · ONE POT

MAKES 12 [2 BITES = 1 SERVING] / PREP TIME: 10 MINUTES / COOK TIME: 20 MINUTES

These bites are convenient to take with you on the go, plus they freeze great.

Nonstick cooking spray, for greasing

¾ cup lactose-free milk or almond milk

⅔ cup mashed unripe bananas (2 medium bananas)

1 large egg

1 teaspoon vanilla extract

3 tablespoons brown sugar

1 teaspoon baking powder

1 teaspoon ground cinnamon

¼ teaspoon salt

2 cups rolled oats

¼ cup semisweet chocolate chips

¼ cup chopped walnuts or pecans (optional)

1. Preheat the oven to 350°F. Grease a 12-cup muffin tin.

2. In a large bowl, mix together the milk, bananas, egg, and vanilla until well combined.

3. Stir in the sugar, baking powder, cinnamon, and salt.

4. Stir in the oats, and mix well.

5. Add the chocolate chips and walnuts (if using).

6. Use a large spoon to divide the oat mixture evenly among the prepared muffin tin cups.

7. Transfer the muffin tin to the oven, and bake for 20 minutes, or until the tops of the bites have browned and all liquid has been absorbed. Remove from the oven.

8. Use a butter knife to loosen the bites, and remove them from the tin. Keep extras in the refrigerator for up to 5 days or a few months in the freezer.

VARIATION TIP: Try using fresh blueberries instead of chocolate chips.

Per Serving (2 bites): Calories: 116; Total Fat: 3g; Saturated Fat: 1g; Cholesterol: 16mg; Sodium: 84mg; Carbohydrates: 20g; Fiber: 2g; Protein: 3g

Denver-Style Omelet

GLUTEN-FREE • 30 MINUTES OR LESS • ONE POT

SERVES 1 / PREP TIME: 5 MINUTES / COOK TIME: 5 MINUTES

Lauren enjoyed an omelet like this one while visiting her grandparents in Denver every summer as a kid. The Denver-Style Omelet has a classic flavor featuring ham, onion, green pepper, and cheese. We use scallions instead of yellow onions to make this recipe low-FODMAP.

3 large eggs

¼ cup chopped smoked ham

2 tablespoons finely chopped scallions, green parts only

2 tablespoons finely chopped green bell pepper

1 teaspoon extra-virgin olive oil or Onion-Infused Oil (page 185)

⅓ cup shredded Cheddar cheese

Pinch salt

Freshly ground black pepper

1. In a medium bowl, whisk together the eggs.
2. Stir in the ham, scallions, and bell pepper.
3. In a medium skillet, heat the oil over medium-low heat.
4. Pour in the egg mixture.
5. Sprinkle the cheese over half the omelet. Cook for 5 minutes, or until the eggs are no longer runny.
6. Fold the omelet in half; the side with the cheese should be the bottom half. Transfer to a plate, and season with salt and pepper.

INGREDIENT TIP: Instead of the scallions, you can use 1 tablespoon dried chives.

VARIATION TIP: If you want to brown the ham and soften the vegetables, you can throw them directly into the skillet. Cook them for a few minutes over medium heat before pouring in the eggs.

FODMAP TIP: Check the ingredients of the smoked ham to make sure there is no added onion or garlic.

Per Serving: Calories: 469; Total Fat: 35g; Saturated Fat: 14g; Cholesterol: 617mg; Sodium: 1042mg; Carbohydrates: 5g; Fiber: 1g; Protein: 34g

Banana Egg Pancakes

VEGETARIAN • 5 INGREDIENTS OR LESS •
30 MINUTES OR LESS • MAKE AHEAD • ONE POT

SERVES 1 / PREP TIME: 2 MINUTES / COOK TIME: 5 MINUTES

You don't need flour to make these low-FODMAP pancakes. These can be whipped up in 5 minutes. Lauren's favorite toppings are a tablespoon of peanut butter and a sprinkle of chocolate chips. A dollop of whipped cream is nice, too.

1 unripe banana

2 large eggs

2 tablespoons rolled oats

¼ teaspoon ground cinnamon

⅛ teaspoon vanilla extract (optional)

1 tablespoon salted butter

1. In a bowl, mash the banana with a fork until smooth.

2. Whisk in the eggs, oats, cinnamon, and vanilla (if using).

3. In large skillet, melt the butter over medium-low heat.

4. Pour the batter into the pan in small circles about 3 inches in diameter. Cook for 3 minutes on the first side, or until lightly browned.

5. Flip the pancakes, and cook for 2 minutes, or until lightly browned. Repeat with the remaining batter. You should end up with 6 mini pancakes.

VARIATION TIP: You can use a tablespoon of oil instead of salted butter, but add a small sprinkle of salt to the batter to help enhance the flavor.

COOKING TIP: For a smoother batter, use your blender.

COOKING TIP: Lauren finds it easiest to make 6 mini pancakes, because larger pancakes can be hard to flip.

Per Serving: Calories: 390; Total Fat: 23g; Saturated Fat: 11g; Cholesterol: 403mg; Sodium: 224mg; Carbohydrates: 35g; Fiber: 4g; Protein: 15g

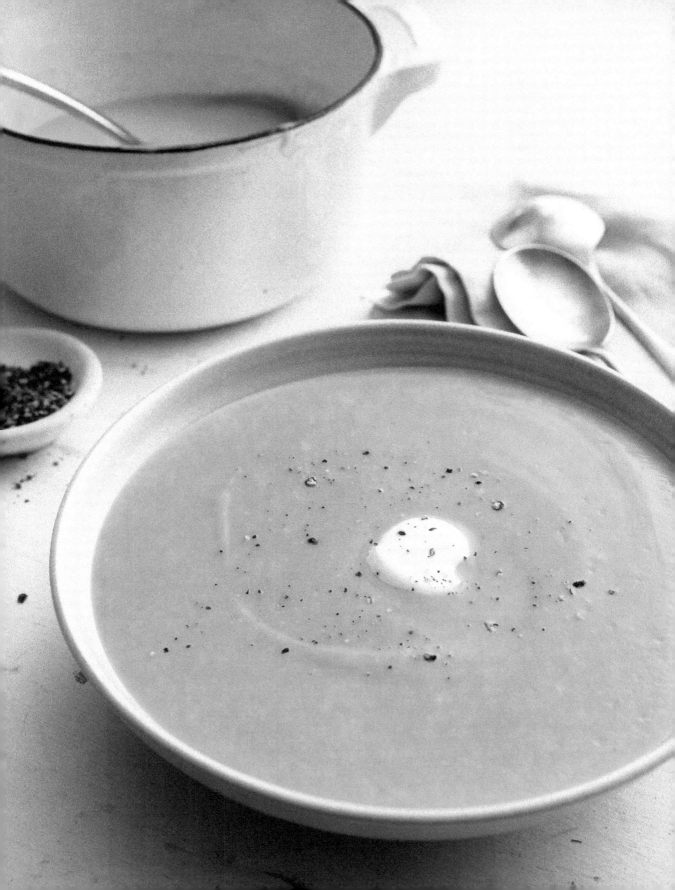

CHAPTER FIVE

Soups, Salads, and Sides

Carrot-Ginger Soup, page 90

Carrot-Ginger Soup

VEGAN · GLUTEN-FREE · ONE POT

SERVES 8 / PREP TIME: 10 MINUTES / COOK TIME: 30 MINUTES

Carrot-ginger is a classic soup that's bursting with flavor. To make it low-FODMAP, we have replaced the onion with fennel bulb, limited the amount of celery, and used our homemade Nourishing Vegetable Broth (page 178). Adding a dollop of a low-FODMAP vegan yogurt on top provides a nice contrast to the spicy ginger.

1 teaspoon extra-virgin olive oil or butter

½ cup coarsely chopped fennel bulb

1 medium celery stalk, coarsely chopped

2 tablespoons grated peeled fresh ginger, plus more as needed

6 cups Nourishing Vegetable Broth (page 178)

6 medium carrots, peeled and coarsely chopped

2 medium yellow potatoes, coarsely chopped

¼ teaspoon freshly ground black pepper, plus more as needed

¼ teaspoon salt, plus more as needed (optional)

½ cup vegan yogurt (optional)

1. In a large pot, heat the oil over medium-high heat.

2. Add the fennel and celery, and sauté for 5 minutes, or until softened.

3. Reduce the heat to medium. Add the ginger, and cook, stirring constantly, for 2 minutes.

4. Add the broth, carrots, potatoes, pepper, and salt (if using). Bring to a boil. Cover, reduce the heat to a simmer, and cook for 15 to 20 minutes, or until the potatoes and carrots are fork-tender.

5. Using an immersion blender or a food processor, purée the soup. Taste, and season with more grated ginger, salt, or pepper, if desired.

6. Serve with extra pepper and a dollop of yogurt (if using) on top.

COOKING TIP: The smaller you chop the carrots and potatoes, the faster the soup will cook.

FODMAP TIP: Carrots and yellow potatoes are free of FODMAPs, so they are good vegetables to fill up on.

Per Serving: Calories: 77; Total Fat: 1g; Saturated Fat: 0g; Cholesterol: 0mg; Sodium: 328mg; Carbohydrates: 16g; Fiber: 3g; Protein: 2g

Curry Lentil Soup

VEGETARIAN · GLUTEN-FREE · MAKE AHEAD · ONE POT

SERVES 4 / PREP TIME: 5 MINUTES / COOK TIME: 30 MINUTES

Everyone needs a go-to lentil soup recipe. The red lentils add a great texture to this soup in addition to so many health benefits. They are high in fiber and a good source of protein and contain antioxidants. The spinach bumps up your iron intake, making this a very well-rounded and wholesome soup.

1 tablespoon extra-virgin olive oil

½ cup chopped leeks, green parts only

1 large carrot, peeled and chopped

2 teaspoons ground coriander

2 teaspoons ground cumin

1 teaspoon ground turmeric

6 cups Nourishing Vegetable Broth (page 178)

½ cup dried red lentils

½ cup quinoa

1 cup chopped spinach

¼ teaspoon salt

Juice of ½ lime

¼ cup sour cream or plain Greek yogurt

¼ cup chopped scallions, green parts only (optional)

¼ cup chopped cilantro (optional)

1. In a large pot, heat the oil over medium-high heat.
2. Add the the leeks, carrot, coriander, cumin, and turmeric, and sauté for 5 minutes, or until softened.
3. Add the broth, lentils, and quinoa. Bring to a boil. Cover, reduce the heat to a simmer, and cook for 30 minutes, or until the lentils and quinoa are tender.
4. Add the spinach, salt, and lime juice.
5. Divide among 4 bowls, and top with a dollop of yogurt, scallions (if using), and cilantro (if using).

VARIATION TIP: Instead of red lentils, you can use 1 cup of canned lentils.

SUBSTITUTION TIP: To make it vegan, use plain coconut yogurt.

Per Serving: Calories: 239; Total Fat: 8g; Saturated Fat: 3g; Cholesterol: 6mg; Sodium: 168mg; Carbohydrates: 32g; Fiber: 10g; Protein: 10g

Comforting Chicken Soup

GLUTEN-FREE · 30 MINUTES OR LESS · MAKE AHEAD · ONE POT

SERVES 4 / PREP TIME: 10 MINUTES / COOK TIME: 20 MINUTES

We've all had days when we want to curl up in a fuzzy blanket with a warm cup of comforting soup. This chicken soup recipe not only cooks quickly and contains only simple ingredients but also is very soothing on your tummy. You will love how moist the chicken tastes from being pulled apart rather than diced. Enjoy it with two fresh slices of traditional sourdough wheat bread and butter.

1 tablespoon extra-virgin olive oil

1 cup chopped leeks, green parts only

2 medium carrots, peeled and chopped

½ celery stalk, chopped

4 cups Nourishing Vegetable Broth
   (page 178) or low-FODMAP
   chicken broth

12 ounces boneless, skinless chicken
   breasts or thighs

½ teaspoon dried rosemary leaves

1. In a large pot, heat the oil over medium-high heat.

2. Add the leeks, carrots, and celery, and sauté for 7 minutes, or until softened.

3. Add the broth, chicken, and rosemary. Bring to a boil, then reduce the heat to a simmer, and cook for 20 minutes.

4. Remove the chicken, and transfer to a cutting board. Using 2 forks, shred into strips.

5. Return the chicken to the pot. Divide the soup among 4 bowls, and serve.

COOKING TIP: Double this recipe, and store it in the freezer for a quick meal.

INGREDIENT TIP: You can use any cut of chicken in this soup or, to save time, use leftover or rotisserie chicken.

Per Serving: Calories: 147; Total Fat: 5g; Saturated Fat: 1g; Cholesterol: 49mg; Sodium: 83mg; Carbohydrates: 6g; Fiber: 1g; Protein: 20g

Caprese Salad

VEGETARIAN • GLUTEN-FREE • 5 INGREDIENTS OR LESS •
30 MINUTES OR LESS • ONE POT

SERVES 4 / PREP TIME: 5 MINUTES

Something magical happens when you combine tomatoes, fresh basil, and cheese. This salad is simple, elegant, and yummy. You can dress it up and serve it with Shrimp Fettuccine (page 137) or dress it down and enjoy with a Tuna Melt (page 132). Either way, it takes only 5 minutes to throw together.

4 ripe tomatoes, each cut into 5 slices

4 ounces bocconcini

2 tablespoons balsamic vinegar

1 tablespoon extra-virgin olive oil

⅓ cup roughly chopped fresh basil or

    1 tablespoon dried basil leaves

Pinch salt

Freshly ground black pepper

1. On a large plate, arrange the tomatoes in a single layer.
2. Cut the bocconcini into 20 pieces. Place 1 piece on each tomato.
3. Drizzle with the vinegar and oil.
4. Top each tomato with basil, and season with salt and pepper.

INGREDIENT TIP: Select vine-ripened tomatoes for a sweet summer tomato flavor.

Per Serving: Calories: 155; Total Fat: 11g; Saturated Fat: 6g; Cholesterol: 25mg; Sodium: 227mg; Carbohydrates: 7g; Fiber: 2g; Protein: 8g

Kale Salad

VEGAN · GLUTEN-FREE · 30 MINUTES OR LESS · MAKE AHEAD · ONE POT

SERVES 4 / PREP TIME: 10 MINUTES

This salad is a nutritious powerhouse packed full of delicious greens. It's like a multivitamin in your bowl, and you get protein and fiber, too. It's a dietitian's dream salad. It will keep for 3 days in the refrigerator and goes well with many of our main dishes, such as the Sun-Dried Tomato and Feta Chicken Sliders (page 144) or Chive-Rubbed Chicken (page 143).

3 large Lacinato kale leaves, stemmed and chopped

1 medium carrot, grated

½ cup chopped red cabbage

⅓ cup chopped fresh cilantro or basil leaves

¼ cup Maple–Balsamic Vinegar Dressing (page 181)

¼ cup sunflower seeds

Pinch salt (optional)

Freshly ground black pepper

1. In a large salad bowl, combine the kale, carrot, cabbage, and cilantro.
2. Drizzle with the dressing, and use your fingers or a salad spoon to gently massage the kale leaves so that they are fully saturated.
3. Top with sunflower seeds, salt (if using), and pepper.

INGREDIENT TIP: Lacinato kale has a milder flavor than curly leaf kale.

VARIATION TIP: Instead of sunflower seeds, you can use roasted pumpkin seeds or walnuts.

Per Serving: Calories: 142; Total Fat: 10g; Saturated Fat: 1g; Cholesterol: 0mg; Sodium: 43mg; Carbohydrates: 11g; Fiber: 2g; Protein: 4g

Classic Coleslaw with a Lime Twist

VEGETARIAN · GLUTEN-FREE · 5 INGREDIENTS OR LESS · 30 MINUTES OR LESS · ONE POT

SERVES 4 / PREP TIME: 15 MINUTES

Premade bag salads are a huge time-saver. In particular, we love bags of coleslaw because they are low-FODMAP and last in the refrigerator for a long time. Also, who doesn't like coleslaw?! Choose a bag of coleslaw that contains white cabbage, red cabbage, and grated carrot with no added onion. This recipe goes really well with Barbecue Pulled Pork (page 151), Chile-Lime DIY Tacos (page 153), and all of the burgers.

½ **cup mayonnaise**

2 **tablespoons freshly squeezed lime juice (about 1 lime)**

1 **tablespoon white sugar**

¼ **teaspoon salt**

4 **cups coleslaw mix**

1. To make the dressing, in a small bowl, mix together the mayonnaise, lime juice, sugar, and salt with a fork until the sugar has completely dissolved.

2. In a medium bowl, combine the coleslaw mix with the dressing.

SUBSTITUTION TIP: To make vegan coleslaw, use vegan mayonnaise.

VARIATION TIP: For a little twist, top the coleslaw with grated lime zest to garnish. Instead of lime juice, use white vinegar, apple cider vinegar, lemon juice, or rice-wine vinegar. Add fresh herbs like parsley, basil, cilantro, or mint to the salad.

Per Serving: Calories: 212; Total Fat: 20g; Saturated Fat: 3g; Cholesterol: 10mg; Sodium: 340mg; Carbohydrates: 8g; Fiber: 2g; Protein: 1g

Greek Quinoa Salad

VEGETARIAN • GLUTEN-FREE • 30 MINUTES OR LESS • MAKE AHEAD • ONE POT

SERVES 6 / PREP TIME: 10 MINUTES / COOK TIME: 15 MINUTES

We love this recipe because it's so easy and healthy. Simply cook the quinoa, chop the vegetables, and mix it together with a simple dressing. It can be a stand-alone meal, or it goes nicely with the Prosciutto-Wrapped Chicken (page 145). Keep the leftovers in the refrigerator, and it will taste even better the next day once the flavors have blended.

1 cup quinoa

3 tablespoons freshly squeezed lemon juice

2 tablespoons Garlic-Infused Oil (page 184) or extra-virgin olive oil

1 teaspoon dried basil or 1 tablespoon minced fresh basil

1 teaspoon dried oregano or 1 tablespoon minced fresh oregano

¼ teaspoon salt

¼ teaspoon freshly ground black pepper

1 cup chopped tomatoes

1 cup chopped cucumber

1 cup chopped red bell pepper

1 cup crumbled feta

½ cup finely chopped scallions, green parts only

½ cup chopped pitted Kalamata olives

1. In a pot, prepare the quinoa according to the package instructions. Transfer to a large bowl, and let cool.

2. To make the dressing, in a small bowl, mix together the lemon juice, oil, basil, oregano, salt, and pepper.

3. Once the quinoa is cool, add the tomatoes, cucumber, bell pepper, feta, scallions, olives, and dressing. Mix well. Taste, and add more seasoning as needed. Store the leftovers in the refrigerator for up to 5 days.

SUBSTITUTION TIP: Make this recipe vegan by using vegan cheese or simply skipping the feta.

Per Serving: Calories: 243; Total Fat: 13g; Saturated Fat: 5g; Cholesterol: 22mg; Sodium: 380mg; Carbohydrates: 24g; Fiber: 3g; Protein: 9g

Sweet Potato Quinoa Cakes

VEGETARIAN • MAKE AHEAD

SERVES 6 [2 CAKES = 1 SERVING] / PREP TIME: 10 MINUTES / COOK TIME: 45 MINUTES

These Sweet Potato Quinoa Cakes are savory, not sweet. They freeze well, which makes this recipe great for batch cooking. Lauren likes eating them with a fried or poached egg on top.

¾ cup quinoa

1 cup grated sweet potato

2 large eggs, beaten

½ cup oat flour

¼ cup pumpkin seeds

¼ cup finely chopped fresh basil leaves

¼ cup finely chopped scallions, green

    parts only

3 tablespoons low-FODMAP flour blend

1 tablespoon almond butter or

    tahini paste

½ tablespoon dried oregano

½ tablespoon red-wine vinegar or

    white vinegar

½ teaspoon salt

1. Preheat the oven to 400°F. Line a sheet pan with parchment paper.

2. In a pot, prepare the quinoa according to the package instructions.

3. Gently press the grated sweet potato in a towel to remove any excess moisture.

4. In a large bowl, combine the cooked quinoa, sweet potato, eggs, oat flour, pumpkin seeds, basil, scallions, flour blend, almond butter, oregano, vinegar, and salt.

5. Shape ¼-cup portions of the mixture into 12 patties, and gently flatten on the prepared sheet pan.

6. Transfer the sheet pan to the oven, and bake for 15 minutes.

7. Flip the cakes, return the sheet pan to the oven, and bake for 10 more minutes, or until lightly browned and firm. Remove from the oven, and let cool for a few minutes. Store in the refrigerator for up to 6 days or in the freezer for up to 3 months.

INGREDIENT TIP: You can make your own oat flour by grinding rolled oats in a food processor or blender.

FODMAP TIP: The low-FODMAP serving size is 3 cakes.

Per Serving (2 cakes): Calories: 227; Total Fat: 8g; Saturated Fat: 1g; Cholesterol: 62mg; Sodium: 232mg; Carbohydrates: 31g; Fiber: 4g; Protein: 9g

Caesar Salad

5 INGREDIENTS OR LESS • 30 MINUTES OR LESS • ONE POT

SERVES 4 / PREP TIME: 10 MINUTES / COOK TIME: 15 MINUTES

Lauren has many fond memories of dinner parties as a child. One of her mom's most popular recipes was Caesar salad with homemade vinaigrette that she prepared in a beautiful wooden salad bowl. Lauren had to create a low-FODMAP variation that was just as delicious. This Caesar salad dressing with Garlic-Infused Oil (page 184) and homemade croutons is one of Lauren's most popular recipes.

4 low-FODMAP bread slices, diced

1½ tablespoons Garlic-Infused Oil (page 184)

1 romaine lettuce head, cut into bite-size pieces

½ cup grated Parmesan cheese

½ cup Caesar Vinaigrette (page 188)

½ cup bacon bits (optional)

1. Preheat oven to 350°F.

2. To make the croutons, in a large bowl, toss the bread with the Garlic-Infused Oil, then place on a sheet pan.

3. Transfer the sheet pan to the oven, and bake, flipping every 5 minutes, for 15 minutes, or until golden brown. Remove from the oven, and let cool.

4. To make the salad, in a large bowl, mix together the lettuce and cheese. Toss with the homemade croutons, vinaigrette, and bacon bits (if using).

VARIATION TIP: Baby kale is a healthy alternative to romaine lettuce.

INGREDIENT TIP: For the croutons, choose bread that is a bit stale (i.e., has been at room temperature for at least a few days).

Per Serving: Calories: 293; Total Fat: 28g; Saturated Fat: 5g; Cholesterol: 11mg; Sodium: 221mg; Carbohydrates: 9g; Fiber: 1g; Protein: 7g

Feta, Tomato, and Spinach Rice

VEGETARIAN · GLUTEN-FREE · 30 MINUTES OR LESS · ONE POT

SERVES 6 / PREP TIME: 5 MINUTES / COOK TIME: 20 MINUTES

Lauren loves making this rice dish as a side for dinner and then taking leftovers to work for lunch. We recommend using the white cooking wine because it helps boost the flavor.

1 tablespoon Onion-Infused Oil
(page 185) or extra-virgin olive oil

1¼ cups basmati rice

2 cups Nourishing Vegetable Broth
(page 178)

¼ cup white cooking wine

2 cups chopped and lightly
packed spinach

1 cup chopped and seeded tomatoes
(2 Roma tomatoes)

1 cup diced feta cheese

½ teaspoon freshly ground black pepper

Pinch salt

1. In a large saucepan, heat the Onion-Infused Oil over medium heat.

2. Once the oil is hot, pour in the rice. Stir and let cook for 2 minutes, or until the rice starts to turn translucent.

3. Pour in the broth and wine. Bring to a boil, then reduce the heat to low. Cover, and simmer for 15 minutes.

4. Stir in the spinach, and cover. Cook for 5 minutes, or until the rice reaches the desired softness. Remove from the heat.

5. Stir in the tomatoes, cheese, pepper, and salt. Keep leftover rice in the refrigerator for up to 1 week or in the freezer for a couple months.

VARIATION TIP: Frozen spinach, kale, or chard can be used instead of fresh spinach. Any long-grain white rice can be used instead of basmati.

Per Serving: Calories: 226; Total Fat: 7g; Saturated Fat: 3g; Cholesterol: 17mg; Sodium: 250mg; Carbohydrates: 34g; Fiber: 1g; Protein: 6g

Cranberry-Quinoa Salad

VEGAN • GLUTEN-FREE • 30 MINUTES OR LESS • MAKE AHEAD • ONE POT

SERVES 8 / PREP TIME: 15 MINUTES / COOK TIME: 15 MINUTES

This dish is a lightly sweet salad that is great for potlucks. Chopped walnuts and cucumber give the salad a nice crunch, and the dark leaves of the scallions boost the flavor without adding any FODMAPs. If you are hesitant to try quinoa, start with this salad.

1 cup quinoa

1 pint cherry tomatoes, halved

1 English cucumber, chopped

1 cup chopped walnuts

½ cup dried cranberries

¼ cup chopped scallions, green
  parts only

½ cup Cranberry Vinaigrette (page 187)

1. In a pot, prepare the quinoa according to the package instructions. Transfer to a large bowl, and let cool for 15 minutes.
2. Add the tomatoes, cucumber, walnuts, cranberries, and scallions.
3. Pour in the dressing, and mix well. Store in an airtight container in the refrigerator for up to 4 days.

COOKING TIP: Use leftover quinoa or prepare the quinoa in advance so it has time to cool and won't cause the green onion to wilt.

FODMAP TIP: A low-FODMAP serving is one-eighth of this recipe. Dried cranberries become high-FODMAP in larger servings.

Per Serving: Calories: 264; Total Fat: 13g; Saturated Fat: 1g; Cholesterol: 0mg; Sodium: 42mg; Carbohydrates: 34g; Fiber: 4g; Protein: 6g

Crispy Parmesan Baby Potatoes

VEGETARIAN • GLUTEN-FREE • 5 INGREDIENTS OR LESS

SERVES 6 / PREP TIME: 5 MINUTES / COOK TIME: 30 MINUTES

Everyone will love this healthy alternative to French fries. Boiling the potatoes is worth the extra step because it ensures they are soft on the inside and nice and crispy on the outside.

1½ pounds baby potatoes

1 tablespoon extra-virgin olive oil

3 tablespoons grated Parmesan cheese, plus more as needed

Pinch salt, plus more as needed

Freshly ground black pepper

1. Preheat the oven to 400°F. Line a sheet pan with parchment paper.
2. Fill a medium saucepan halfway with water, and bring to a boil.
3. Add the potatoes, reduce the heat to low, and simmer for 10 minutes.
4. Drain the potatoes in a colander. Rinse with cold water, and dry. Chop in half. If there are any extra-large baby potatoes, quarter them instead.
5. In a large bowl, toss the potatoes with the oil and cheese, and season with the salt and pepper. Pour onto the prepared sheet pan.
6. Transfer the sheet pan to the oven, and bake, flipping halfway through, for 20 minutes, or until browned. Remove from the oven.
7. Add more cheese, pepper, or salt as desired. Leftovers will keep in the refrigerator for up to 5 days.

INGREDIENT TIP: Baby potatoes are convenient because they do not need to be peeled and are often sold prewashed. If you would rather use large yellow potatoes, scrub them clean, and chop them into bite-size pieces.

VARIATION TIP: Any color baby potatoes can be used. Keep an eye out in your grocery store for a bag of multicolor potatoes.

Per Serving: Calories: 122; Total Fat: 3g; Saturated Fat: 1g; Cholesterol: 3mg; Sodium: 77mg; Carbohydrates: 20g; Fiber: 3g; Protein: 4g

Pomegranate, Poppy Seed, and Spinach Salad

**VEGETARIAN · GLUTEN-FREE · 5 INGREDIENTS OR LESS ·
30 MINUTES OR LESS · ONE POT**

SERVES 4 / PREP TIME: 5 MINUTES

Your whole family will love this sweet salad. Lauren's cousin once warmly referred to this as "dessert salad" because he thinks it is so sweet and tasty. It is especially nice to serve during December with its beautiful red and green colors.

4 ounces baby spinach

½ cup crumbled goat cheese

½ cup pomegranate seeds

⅓ cup walnut pieces

¼ cup Poppy Seed Salad Dressing
(page 190)

In a large bowl, toss the spinach with the goat cheese, pomegranate seeds, walnuts, and dressing. Serve immediately.

SUBSTITUTION TIP: Use a vegan cheese instead of goat cheese to make this recipe vegan.

VARIATION TIP: Try diced mozzarella or Swiss cheese instead of crumbled goat cheese. Sliced strawberries are also a great alternative to pomegranate seeds.

Per Serving: Calories: 242; Total Fat: 20g; Saturated Fat: 4g; Cholesterol: 5mg; Sodium: 224mg; Carbohydrates: 11g; Fiber: 2g; Protein: 5g

Cajun-Spiced Root Vegetable Fries

VEGAN · GLUTEN-FREE · ONE POT

SERVES 4 / PREP TIME: 10 MINUTES / COOK TIME: 30 MINUTES

The combination of the four different root vegetables creates an incredible variety of textures and flavors to these hand-cut fries. Baked fries can be just as crispy as the deep-fried alternatives, and they are way healthier. We spiced these up with our homemade Cajun seasoning mix.

2 cups sweet potato, cut into sticks

1 medium yellow or red potato, cut into sticks

1 large carrot, cut into sticks

1 large parsnip, cut into sticks

2 tablespoons Garlic-Infused Oil (page 184) or extra-virgin olive oil

2 tablespoons Cajun Spice Mix (page 186)

Pinch salt

Freshly ground black pepper

1. Preheat the oven to 425°F. Line a large sheet pan with parchment paper.
2. Dry the sweet potato, potato, carrot, and parsnip with a paper towel to remove excess starch and moisture. Place in a large bowl, and toss with the oil.
3. Sprinkle on the Cajun Spice Mix, and toss to mix. Season with salt and pepper. Place in a single layer on the prepared sheet pan.
4. Transfer the sheet pan to the oven, and bake for 15 minutes.
5. Flip the fries, return the sheet pan to the oven, and bake for 10 to 15 minutes, or until crispy and browned.

Per Serving: Calories: 145; Total Fat: 5g; Saturated Fat: 1g; Cholesterol: 0mg; Sodium: 124mg; Carbohydrates: 25g; Fiber: 5g; Protein: 2g

Warm Roasted Vegetable Salad

VEGAN · GLUTEN-FREE

SERVES 6 / PREP TIME: 10 MINUTES / COOK TIME: 30 MINUTES

This salad is a nice alternative to a leafy green salad in the wintertime. We love how this bowl of quinoa is topped with roasted vegetables, chopped greens, and seeds, then drizzled with dressing. Lauren prefers to roast the vegetables for the entire 30 minutes so that they get nicely charred.

1 cup quinoa

2 cups chopped broccoli

2 cups chopped (½ inch) yellow or red potatoes

2 cups cut (bite-size) green beans

1½ tablespoons extra-virgin olive oil

Pinch salt

Freshly ground black pepper

1 cup chopped baby spinach or greens

¼ cup finely chopped scallions, green parts only

1 recipe Maple–Balsamic Vinegar Dressing (page 181)

¼ cup pumpkin seeds or sunflower seeds

1. Preheat the oven to 400°F. Line a large sheet pan with parchment paper.

2. In a pot, prepare the quinoa according to the package instructions.

3. In a bowl, toss the broccoli, potatoes, and green beans with the oil. Spread onto the prepared sheet pan. Season with the salt and pepper.

4. Transfer the sheet pan to the oven, and roast for 15 minutes.

5. Flip the vegetables, return the sheet pan to the oven, and roast for 5 to 15 minutes (more or less time depending on how charred you want the vegetables).

6. To serve, fill a bowl with the quinoa, and top with the roasted vegetables, spinach, and scallions. Drizzle the dressing on top, add the seeds, and mix. Store leftovers in an airtight container in the refrigerator for up to 5 days.

VARIATION TIP: You can swap the broccoli and green beans with any variation of carrots and parsnips. The quinoa can be cooked in vegetable broth to increase the flavor. Brown rice is a nice alternative to quinoa. Add tofu or a cup of drained and rinsed chickpeas for a protein boost and to make this salad into a stand-alone meal.

Per Serving: Calories: 286; Total Fat: 14g; Saturated Fat: 2g; Cholesterol: 0mg; Sodium: 57mg; Carbohydrates: 34g; Fiber: 6g; Protein: 8g

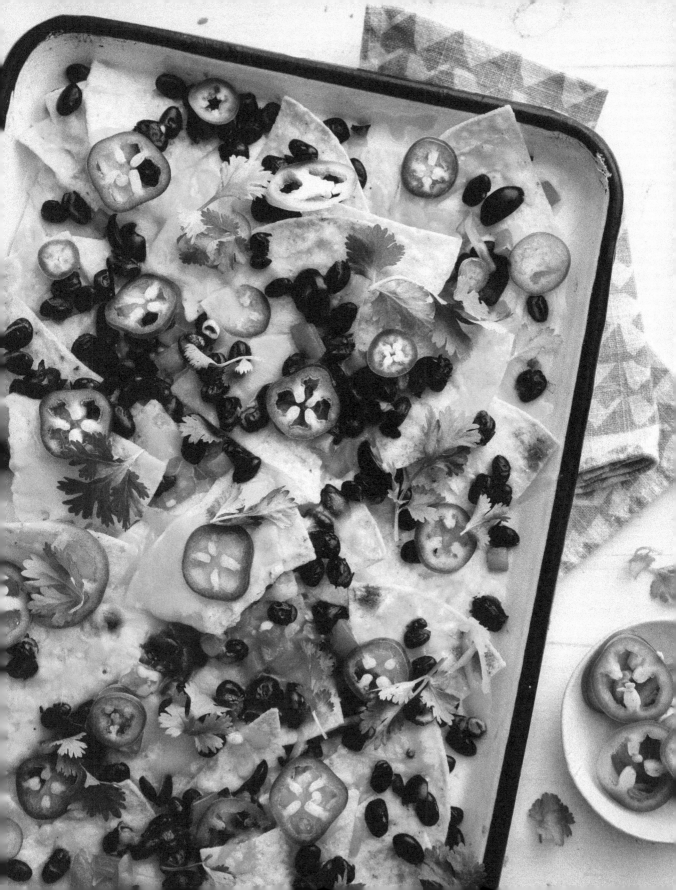

CHAPTER SIX

Meatless Mains

Bell Pepper Mini Pizzas

**VEGETARIAN · GLUTEN-FREE · 5 INGREDIENTS OR LESS ·
30 MINUTES OR LESS · ONE POT**

SERVES 4 / PREP TIME: 5 MINUTES / COOK TIME: 10 MINUTES

Craving pizza? Try out these bell pepper mini pizzas. They are much easier to make than pizza made with dough, and you can add any low-FODMAP toppings you like to make these your own. Lauren likes to top them with sliced cherry tomatoes and a sprinkle of grated Parmesan cheese.

4 red bell peppers

⅓ cup plain tomato sauce

⅔ cup shredded mozzarella cheese

1½ teaspoons dried basil (optional)

1½ teaspoons dried oregano (optional)

1. Preheat the oven to 350°F. Line a sheet pan with parchment paper.
2. Stand each bell pepper upright, and cut along the ridges of the peppers, from top to bottom, slicing each pepper into 4 pieces. Remove the stem, seeds, and any white flesh on the inside of the peppers.
3. Place the pepper slices skin-side down on the prepared sheet pan.
4. Divide the tomato sauce among the pepper slices and then sprinkle with mozzarella.
5. Sprinkle on the basil and oregano (if using).
6. Transfer the sheet pan to the oven, and bake for 8 to 10 minutes, or until the cheese has fully melted and the peppers have softened. Remove from the oven.

COOKING TIP: The average bell pepper has 4 ridges and will be cut into 4 pieces when you cut along the ridges.

Per Serving: Calories: 118; Total Fat: 6g; Saturated Fat: 3g; Cholesterol: 19mg; Sodium: 190mg; Carbohydrates: 11g; Fiber: 2g; Protein: 7g

Broccoli and Cheese Frittata

VEGETARIAN · GLUTEN-FREE · MAKE AHEAD · ONE POT

SERVES 6 / PREP TIME: 10 MINUTES / COOK TIME: 35 MINUTES

A baked frittata is perfect for anyone who finds that their omelets often turn into scrambled eggs. Broccoli and Cheddar cheese are a winning combination. Enjoy this frittata for dinner, breakfast, or lunch. Leftovers can be eaten hot or cold.

Nonstick cooking spray, for greasing

2 cups chopped broccoli

1 cup chopped spinach

1 cup shredded Cheddar cheese

½ cup finely chopped scallions, green parts only

12 large eggs

1 teaspoon dried oregano or 2 teaspoons fresh minced oregano

½ teaspoon freshly ground black pepper

1. Preheat the oven to 350°F. Grease a glass 9-by-13-inch baking dish.

2. Scatter the broccoli, spinach, cheese, and scallions evenly in the baking dish.

3. Crack the eggs into a large bowl, and whisk in the oregano and pepper.

4. Pour the whisked eggs over the vegetables.

5. Transfer the baking dish to the oven, and bake for about 35 minutes, or until the eggs are puffed and set. The center of the frittata should jiggle just a bit when you give it a gentle shake. Remove from the oven, and let cool for 5 minutes.

6. Slice the frittata into pieces, and serve warm. Store leftover slices in an airtight container in the refrigerator for up to 4 days.

COOKING TIP: Grease the baking dish very well, including all four sides. Otherwise, cleanup can be a hassle.

VARIATION TIP: If you would prefer the broccoli to be soft instead of crunchy, steam it for 3 minutes, and pat it dry, before adding it to the baking dish.

Per Serving: Calories: 234; Total Fat: 16g; Saturated Fat: 7g; Cholesterol: 362mg; Sodium: 272mg; Carbohydrates: 4g; Fiber: 1g; Protein: 19g

Curry Egg Salad Sandwich

VEGETARIAN · 30 MINUTES OR LESS · ONE POT · MAKE AHEAD

SERVES 1 / PREP TIME: 5 MINUTES / COOK TIME: 15 MINUTES

Years ago, Lauren would always get curry-spiced egg salad sandwiches from the Cornerstone Cafe in Guelph, Ontario. When she moved to Toronto, she made her own IBS-friendly version at home. This recipe optimizes taste and nutrition by using half mayonnaise and half Greek yogurt. Just remember a small amount of curry powder adds a lot of flavor, and you can add extra if desired.

2 large eggs

2 tablespoons finely chopped scallions, green parts only

1 tablespoon mayonnaise

1 tablespoon lactose-free plain Greek yogurt

⅛ teaspoon curry powder

2 low-FODMAP bread slices, lightly toasted

Salt

Freshly ground black pepper

1. Fill a bowl with ice water. In a small saucepan, cover the eggs with cold water. Bring to a rolling boil over medium-high heat, and cook for 15 minutes. Drain, and place the eggs in the bowl of ice water to cool, then peel and chop.

2. In a small bowl, mix together the eggs, scallions, mayonnaise, yogurt, and curry powder.

3. Divide the egg mixture between the pieces of toast. Season with salt and pepper.

VARIATION TIP: Two other favorite ways to serve these curried eggs are open-faced with baby spinach and tomato slices, or on top of cucumber slices.

COOKING TIP: Hardboiled eggs will last in the refrigerator for up to 7 days.

FODMAP TIP: When purchasing curry powder, avoid any brands that contain garlic or onion. Lauren often uses Dion brand curry powder.

Per Serving: Calories: 367; Total Fat: 22g; Saturated Fat: 5g; Cholesterol: 378mg; Sodium: 443mg; Carbohydrates: 26g; Fiber: 6g; Protein: 20g

Cheesy Italian Baked Eggs

VEGETARIAN • 30 MINUTES OR LESS • ONE POT

SERVES 3 / PREP TIME: 10 MINUTES / COOK TIME: 15 MINUTES

Lauren's favorite way to enjoy this dish is by dipping sourdough bread slices into the baked eggs. The sourdough pairs nicely with the acidic tomato sauce. The eggs and cheese add an excellent source of protein.

Extra-virgin olive oil, for greasing

2 cups tomato sauce

¾ cup chopped stemmed spinach

6 large eggs

½ cup shredded mozzarella cheese

1 tablespoon grated Parmesan
    cheese (optional)

¼ teaspoon dried basil

6 sourdough bread slices or other
    low-FODMAP bread

1. Preheat the oven to 400°F. Grease a glass 9-by-13-inch baking dish.

2. In small saucepan, heat the tomato sauce over medium heat.

3. Stir the spinach into the tomato sauce, and cook for 2 minutes, or until the spinach has wilted. Pour into the prepared baking dish.

4. Use a large spoon to make an egg-size hole in the sauce. Crack an egg into the hole. Repeat with the remaining eggs.

5. Sprinkle the mozzarella cheese onto the tomato sauce around the eggs.

6. Sprinkle the Parmesan cheese (if using) and basil over the entire dish.

7. Transfer the baking dish to the oven, and bake for 10 minutes, or until the eggs are solid and no longer runny. Remove from the oven. Serve with slices of sourdough. Store leftovers in an airtight container in the refrigerator for up to 4 days.

VARIATION TIP: Frozen spinach can be used instead of fresh. Defrost the spinach, and drain off any liquid that is released before chopping and adding to the tomato sauce.

Per Serving: Calories: 409; Total Fat: 17g; Saturated Fat: 7g; Cholesterol: 389mg; Sodium: 955mg; Carbohydrates: 41g; Fiber: 4g; Protein: 26g

Mushroom Quinoa Burgers

VEGETARIAN • MAKE AHEAD

SERVES 4 / PREP TIME: 15 MINUTES / COOK TIME: 20 MINUTES

The combination of mushrooms and smoked Cheddar makes this a veggie burger that even hardcore carnivores love. You may be surprised to see mushrooms in this recipe. Luckily for us, not all mushrooms are high-FODMAP. Canned mushrooms are lower in FODMAPs than other mushrooms.

¼ cup quinoa

1 cup finely chopped canned mushrooms

1 large egg

½ cup chopped scallions, green

parts only

⅓ cup shredded smoked Cheddar cheese

¼ cup finely chopped walnuts

¼ cup gluten-free bread crumbs

1½ teaspoons soy sauce

1. In a pot, prepare the quinoa according to the package instructions.
2. Preheat the oven to 400°F. Line a sheet pan with parchment paper.
3. Remove most of the moisture from the mushrooms by wrapping them in paper towels and squeezing the water out. They should be relatively dry. Then chop them very finely.
4. In a large bowl, beat the egg with a fork.
5. Add the mushrooms, scallions, cheese, walnuts, bread crumbs, and soy sauce.
6. Shape ½-cup portions of the mixture into 4 (1-inch-thick) patties. Place on the prepared sheet pan, leaving 1 inch between patties.
7. Transfer the sheet pan to the oven, and bake for 8 minutes per side, or until browned and crispy. Remove from the oven.

COOKING TIP: To save time, prepare the quinoa in advance, or use leftover quinoa. These burgers freeze well and will keep in the freezer for 3 months.

FODMAP TIP: A low-FODMAP serving is 1 burger per meal.

Per Serving: Calories: 175; Total Fat: 10g; Saturated Fat: 3g; Cholesterol: 56mg; Sodium: 192mg; Carbohydrates: 15g; Fiber: 2g; Protein: 8g

Crispy Tofu

VEGAN • 5 INGREDIENTS OR LESS • 30 MINUTES OR LESS • ONE POT

SERVES 4 / PREP TIME: 5 MINUTES / COOK TIME: 12 MINUTES

The great thing about tofu is that it absorbs the flavors you combine it with. When tofu is pressed to remove the moisture, it behaves like a sponge and absorbs even more sauce. Sear the sides and add a splash of soy sauce to make this dish an easy addition to many meatless meals. To jazz it up, try it with the Creamy Dipping Duo (page 182).

1 pound extra-firm tofu, cut into 24 pieces

1 tablespoon sesame oil or coconut oil

1 tablespoon soy sauce

1. Wrap the tofu with a clean tea towel or a few sheets of paper towel, and firmly squeeze out the moisture with your hands for about 1 minute. Rewrap the tofu, and press it again.

2. In a large nonstick skillet, heat the oil over medium heat.

3. Add the tofu in a single layer.

4. Once the bottom has browned, tip the tofu over, and sear the next side. It will take about 12 minutes to brown all sides of the tofu. Remove from the heat.

5. Splash the tofu evenly with the soy sauce.

COOKING TIP: The trick to preventing tofu from sticking is to allow it to brown and get crispy on the bottom before turning it. If you turn it too early, it will stick.

INGREDIENT TIP: Use oil with a high smoke point, such as coconut or sesame. Olive oil will burn.

FODMAP TIP: Extra-firm tofu is lower in FODMAPs than softer varieties like firm and silken.

Per Serving: Calories: 135; Total Fat: 10g; Saturated Fat: 4g; Cholesterol: 0mg; Sodium: 186mg; Carbohydrates: 3g; Fiber: 1g; Protein: 12g

Tofu Noodle Bowl

VEGAN • 30 MINUTES OR LESS • ONE POT

SERVES 2 / PREP TIME: 18 MINUTES / COOK TIME: 12 MINUTES

This beautiful noodle bowl is Audrey's all-time favorite vegan dish. She loves serving it with Goddess Dressing (page 179), which is a low-FODMAP adaptation of the Glory Bowl Dressing from Whitewater Cooks. It is so good you could drink it with a straw!

6 ounces thin rice noodles

2 packed cups baby spinach leaves

1 cup shredded or spiralized carrot

½ recipe Crispy Tofu (page 113)

¼ cup Goddess Dressing (page 179)

¼ cup unsalted peanuts

2 teaspoons maple syrup (optional)

1. In a pot, prepare the rice noodles according to the package instructions. Divide between 2 bowls.

2. Add the spinach, carrot, and tofu.

3. Top with the dressing, peanuts, and maple syrup (if using).

COOKING TIP: Place the spinach on top of the rice noodles when they are very hot so the heat wilts the spinach.

VARIATION TIP: Use shredded cucumber, red bell pepper, or a cup of broccoli instead of carrots or spinach.

Per Serving: Calories: 644; Total Fat: 21g; Saturated Fat: 6g; Cholesterol: 0mg; Sodium: 752mg; Carbohydrates: 88g; Fiber: 8g; Protein: 26g

Thai Peanut Stir-Fry

VEGAN · 30 MINUTES OR LESS

SERVES 4 / PREP TIME: 15 MINUTES / COOK TIME: 10 MINUTES

Thailand is one of Audrey's favorite countries to visit. Unfortunately, many Thai dishes contain high-FODMAP ingredients. Here's a healthy Thai-inspired stir-fry that makes for a quick and easy dinner. Serve it with either rice or rice noodles while dreaming of palm tree-lined white sandy beaches.

½ cup canned coconut milk

¼ cup natural peanut butter

2 tablespoons soy sauce

2 tablespoons brown sugar

1 tablespoon minced peeled fresh ginger
   or 1 teaspoon ground ginger

15 large Thai basil leaves, finely
   chopped (optional)

2 carrots, peeled and chopped
   ¼-inch thick

2 red bell peppers, chopped

2 cups chopped broccoli florets

¼ cup water

1 recipe Crispy Tofu (page 113)

¼ cup sliced scallions, green parts only

1. To make the sauce, in a food processor, combine the coconut milk, peanut butter, soy sauce, sugar, ginger, and basil (if using). Blend on medium for 1 minute, or until smooth.

2. To make the stir fry, remove the tofu from the skillet you cooked it in, and add the carrots, bell peppers, broccoli, and water to the skillet. Cover, and cook over medium-high heat for 5 minutes, or until the vegetables are lightly steamed and fork-tender.

3. Add the tofu, sauce, and scallions to the skillet, and stir to combine. Remove from the heat.

COOKING TIP: Double the sauce to keep for the next time you make this dish.

VARIATION TIP: Instead of broccoli, use 2 cups chopped green beans or bok choy.

FODMAP TIP: Broccoli heads are lower in FODMAPs than the stems, so use mostly heads for this recipe.

Per Serving: Calories: 375; Total Fat: 26g; Saturated Fat: 12g; Cholesterol: 0mg; Sodium: 586mg; Carbohydrates: 24g; Fiber: 6g; Protein: 21g

Tofu BLT

VEGAN • 30 MINUTES OR LESS • ONE POT

SERVES 2 / PREP TIME: 10 MINUTES / COOK TIME: 10 MINUTES

Audrey and her husband, Dave, discovered this sandwich at a vegetarian restaurant in Edmonton about 20 years ago. It's now been a weekend lunch staple for just as long. The trick to making the tofu taste like bacon is to slice it very thin, season it with soy sauce, and fry it until it is brown and crispy. Serve the sandwich with a side of sliced vegetables like cucumber and carrots.

8 ounces extra-firm tofu, cut into 8 slices

2 tablespoons soy sauce

1 tablespoon maple syrup or brown sugar

2 tablespoons coconut oil

4 low-FODMAP bread slices, toasted

1 tablespoon vegan mayonnaise

1 tablespoon Dijon mustard (optional)

1 tomato, thinly sliced

4 lettuce leaves

Freshly ground black pepper

1. Wrap the tofu with a clean tea towel or a few sheets of paper towel, and firmly squeeze out the moisture with your hands for about 1 minute. Rewrap the tofu, and press it again.

2. In a dish with a large flat surface area, combine the soy sauce and maple syrup. Stir well.

3. Lay the tofu in the dish, and turn each slice so all surfaces are coated. Let marinate for 5 minutes or as long as 20 minutes.

4. In a large skillet, heat the oil over medium-high heat.

5. Place the tofu in the pan in a single layer. Sauté for 4 minutes per side, or until golden brown and crispy.

6. Spread the mayonnaise and mustard (if using) onto the toast, then top with the tomato, lettuce, and tofu. Season with pepper.

VARIATION TIP: You can add a slice of vegan cheese (or Cheddar cheese, if you eat it) to each sandwich for extra flavor.

FODMAP TIP: Choose extra-firm tofu as it has a meatier texture and is lower in FODMAPs than the softer types.

Per Serving: Calories: 431; Total Fat: 25g; Saturated Fat: 13g; Cholesterol: 2mg; Sodium: 1259mg; Carbohydrates: 37g; Fiber: 5g; Protein: 20g

Chickpea, Feta, and Tofu Salad

VEGETARIAN · GLUTEN-FREE · 30 MINUTES OR LESS · ONE POT

SERVES 4 / PREP TIME: 15 MINUTES / COOK TIME: 10 MINUTES

This salad is topped with a lovely medley of chickpeas, feta, and crispy tofu. It makes a nice light dinner salad and can be enjoyed with quinoa or traditional sourdough bread.

1 teaspoon sunflower oil

½ teaspoon salt, divided

½ pound extra-firm tofu, cut into
   ½-inch dice

¼ cup extra-virgin olive oil

Juice of 1 lemon

¼ teaspoon salt

Freshly ground black pepper

8 romaine lettuce leaves, chopped

3 tomatoes, chopped

1 cucumber, chopped

½ cup chopped scallions, green
   parts only

½ cup chopped fresh parsley

1 cup feta cheese, diced

½ cup canned chickpeas, drained
   and rinsed

1. In a medium bowl, combine the sunflower oil and ¼ teaspoon of salt, and mix well.

2. Add the tofu, and mix gently so that the mixture covers the tofu evenly.

3. Heat a large nonstick skillet over medium heat.

4. Add the tofu, and sauté, turning occasionally, for 10 minutes, or until each side is golden brown.

5. To make the dressing, in a medium bowl, mix together the olive oil, lemon juice, and remaining ¼ teaspoon salt with a fork until smooth. Season with pepper.

6. In a large salad bowl, combine the lettuce, tomatoes, cucumber, scallions, and parsley.

7. Add the dressing to the salad, and toss gently. Top with the tofu, cheese, and chickpeas.

VARIATION TIP: If you prefer poultry, you can substitute chicken for the tofu in this recipe.

Per Serving: Calories: 343; Total Fat: 26g; Saturated Fat: 8g; Cholesterol: 33mg; Sodium: 538mg; Carbohydrates: 18g; Fiber: 4g; Protein: 15g

Loaded Nachos

VEGETARIAN · GLUTEN-FREE · 30 MINUTES OR LESS · ONE POT

SERVES 2 / PREP TIME: 10 MINUTES / COOK TIME: 2 MINUTES

Thank goodness you can still enjoy nachos on the low-FODMAP diet. Here's a quick recipe that definitely won't leave you feeling deprived. Alternatively, you can scale it down and just have Fresh Cut Salsa (page 177) and tortilla chips. Both are great snacks.

6 ounces corn tortilla chips

½ cup canned black beans, drained and rinsed

½ tomato, finely chopped

½ cup chopped pitted Kalamata olives

1 cup shredded Cheddar cheese

½ recipe Fresh Cut Salsa (page 177)

¼ cup lactose-free sour cream

¼ cup chopped scallions, green parts only

¼ cup chopped cilantro (optional)

Jalapeño pepper slices (optional)

1. Set the oven to broil. Line a sheet pan with parchment paper.
2. Spread the chips evenly onto the prepared sheet pan.
3. Top with the beans, tomato, olives, and cheese.
4. Transfer the sheet pan to the oven, and broil for 2 minutes, or until the cheese is melted and bubbly. Remove from the oven.
5. Top with the salsa, sour cream, scallions, cilantro (if using), and jalapeño peppers (if using).

VARIATION TIP: If you add jalapeño peppers, be mindful that they can be a digestive trigger for some people.

COOKING TIP: Label and store the leftover black beans in the freezer in ¼-cup or ½-cup portions.

Per Serving: Calories: 810; Total Fat: 48g; Saturated Fat: 17g; Cholesterol: 70mg; Sodium: 997mg; Carbohydrates: 74g; Fiber: 12g; Protein: 26g

Lentil Shepherd's Pie

VEGETARIAN · GLUTEN-FREE · MAKE AHEAD

SERVES 4 / PREP TIME: 15 MINUTES / COOK TIME: 50 MINUTES

In Audrey's household, mashed potatoes are affectionately referred to as cloud fluff. Here, the fluffiness of the potatoes is nicely balanced with the hearty lentil filling. Crisscross the top layer with a fork and then set the oven on broil for the last minute to make a crunchy top.

FOR THE MASHED POTATOES

1½ pounds yellow potatoes, quartered
   (6 medium potatoes)

4 tablespoons (½ stick) butter
   or margarine

¼ cup cream or lactose-free milk

Pinch salt

FOR THE FILLING

1 tablespoon extra-virgin olive oil

1 cup chopped leeks, green parts only

3 carrots, peeled and finely chopped

1 cup Nourishing Vegetable Broth
   (page 178), divided

1 (15-ounce) can lentils, drained
   and rinsed

1 teaspoon dried thyme

Pinch salt

Freshly ground black pepper

TO MAKE THE MASHED POTATOES

1. In a large pot, cover the potatoes with water, and bring to a boil over medium-high heat. Cook for 20 minutes, or until you can easily insert a knife. Drain with a colander.

2. Return the potatoes to the pot, and mash with a potato masher.

3. Add the butter and cream. Mix well, and season with salt.

TO MAKE THE FILLING

1. Preheat the oven to 425°F.

2. In a large skillet, heat the oil over medium heat.

3. Add the leeks and carrot, cook for 2 minutes, then pour in ½ cup of broth. Cook for 8 minutes, uncovered, or until the carrots are soft.

4. Add the lentils and thyme.

> CONTINUED ON NEXT PAGE

5. In a small bowl, mix the remaining ½ cup of broth with 2 tablespoons of mashed potatoes, and add to the skillet. Mash the vegetable-lentil mixture a few times with the potato masher and then stir to thicken it. Season with the salt and pepper.

6. Pour the filling into an 8-inch square baking dish. Top with the remaining mashed potatoes. Gently press the potatoes until flat. Use a fork to make a crisscross pattern on the top.

7. Transfer the baking dish to the oven, bake for 15 minutes, then set the oven to broil. Cook for 3 minutes, or until the top is brown and crispy.

FODMAP TIP: You can use regular cream since the lactose content for this amount is low-FODMAP. A low-FODMAP serving is one-quarter of the recipe.

Per Serving: Calories: 376; Total Fat: 16g; Saturated Fat: 8g; Cholesterol: 32mg; Sodium: 175mg; Carbohydrates: 50g; Fiber: 12g; Protein: 11g

Lentil-Squash Stew

VEGAN · GLUTEN-FREE · MAKE AHEAD · ONE POT

SERVES 10 / PREP TIME: 10 MINUTES / COOK TIME: 35 MINUTES

This stew features kabocha squash, which is also known as Japanese pumpkin. This type of squash doesn't contain any FODMAPs, and it has a creamier texture. One of the best features of this stew is how well it freezes. When you cook a big batch, you can freeze the extras for up to 3 months! Having a premade healthy low-FODMAP meal in your freezer is a huge time-saver for busy days.

1 tablespoon extra-virgin olive oil

1½ cups finely chopped fennel bulb

8 cups diced (1-inch) peeled
   kabocha squash

½ cup finely chopped scallions, green
   parts only

3 cups Nourishing Vegetable Broth
   (page 178)

2 cups canned lentils, drained and rinsed

1 (14½-ounce) can diced tomatoes

1 (13½-ounce) can full-fat coconut milk

3 tablespoons tomato paste

1½ teaspoons ground cumin

1 teaspoon ground turmeric

1 teaspoon ancho chile powder
   (no garlic)

2 teaspoons apple cider
   vinegar (optional)

Salt

Freshly ground black pepper

1. In a large saucepot, heat the oil over medium heat.

2. Add the fennel, and cook for 3 minutes, then stir in the squash and scallions, and cook for 2 minutes, or until the fennel has slightly softened.

3. Pour in the broth, lentils, diced tomatoes and their juices, coconut milk, tomato paste, cumin, turmeric, and chile powder. Bring to a boil, then reduce the heat to medium-low, and simmer for 30 minutes, or until the squash is soft. Remove from the heat.

4. Add the apple cider vinegar (if using). Once cooled, transfer to a blender (or use an immersion blender), and blend the soup in 2-second increments until the desired thickness is achieved; avoid overblending. Season with salt and pepper. Store in an airtight container in the refrigerator for up to 5 days or in the freezer for up to 3 months.

> CONTINUED ON NEXT PAGE

VARIATION TIP: After the soup has been blended, you can add some greens or herbs. A cup of chopped spinach adds extra nutrition. Or try ½ cup fresh parsley for a fresh flavor. This stew also tastes delicious with Cheddar cheese (or a vegan cheese) sprinkled on top.

COOKING TIP: Blending is optional but recommended because it helps thicken the soup. An immersion blender is easiest for soups. Blend before adding any optional greens, herbs, or cheese.

INGREDIENT TIP: You will be able to get approximately 8 cups of chopped squash from a 3-pound kabocha squash.

Per Serving: Calories: 294; Total Fat: 21g; Saturated Fat: 17g; Cholesterol: 0mg; Sodium: 42mg; Carbohydrates: 25g; Fiber: 7g; Protein: 7g

Roasted Red Pepper Hippy Bowl

VEGETARIAN • GLUTEN-FREE • 30 MINUTES OR LESS

SERVES 4 / PREP TIME: 15 MINUTES / COOK TIME: 15 MINUTES

The sauce is the highlight of this dish. You will likely bookmark this one just for the sauce alone. To add some more "hippy" to your plate, enjoy it with wilted spinach, a mixed green salad, or roasted vegetables like parsnips and carrots.

¾ cup rice, any type

1 (10-ounce) jar roasted red peppers or
   2 whole roasted peppers

¾ cup walnuts

3 tablespoons extra-virgin olive oil

2 tablespoons lightly packed
   brown sugar

1 teaspoon freshly ground black pepper

1 teaspoon ground cumin

½ teaspoon salt

½ teaspoon smoked or regular paprika

1 (15-ounce) can lentils, drained
   and rinsed

1 tablespoon Garlic-Infused Oil
   (page 184) or extra-virgin olive
   oil (optional)

½ cup crumbled feta cheese

Freshly ground black pepper

1. In a pot, prepare the rice according to the package instructions.

2. To make the sauce, in a food processor, combine the peppers, walnuts, olive oil, sugar, pepper, cumin, salt, and paprika. Blend until smooth like the texture of hummus.

3. In a large serving bowl, gently combine the lentils, cooked rice, and oil (if using).

4. Divide the lentils and rice among 4 serving bowls, add a generous dollop of sauce, then top with feta, and season with pepper.

VARIATION TIP: Substitute the lentils with 1 can of either canned chickpeas or black beans. Quinoa can replace the rice.

COOKING TIP: Double the roasted red pepper sauce recipe—we guarantee that you will find a million uses for it. You can store extra sauce in an airtight container in the refrigerator for 2 weeks or freeze for up to 3 months.

Per Serving: Calories: 563; Total Fat: 32g; Saturated Fat: 6g; Cholesterol: 17mg; Sodium: 475mg; Carbohydrates: 58g; Fiber: 13g; Protein: 16g

Lentil-Walnut Lettuce Wraps

VEGAN · GLUTEN-FREE · 30 MINUTES OR LESS · MAKE AHEAD · ONE POT

SERVES 4 / PREP TIME: 20 MINUTES

These wraps will convince you that lentils and walnuts make for a beautiful match. Audrey prefers the lightness of wrapping them with a crispy lettuce leaf instead of a corn tortilla, but you can choose what you like best. These wraps pair nicely with rice, quinoa, or a baked potato.

1 (15-ounce) can lentils, drained
   and rinsed

1 cup walnut pieces

1 tablespoon Garlic-Infused Oil
   (page 184) or extra-virgin olive oil

1½ teaspoons ground cumin

½ teaspoon dried oregano

½ teaspoon chili powder (no garlic)

½ teaspoon salt

1 red bell pepper, finely chopped

¼ cup chopped scallions, green
   parts only

¼ cup chopped fresh cilantro

½ cup shredded vegan cheese (optional)

1 small lettuce head

Vegan mayonnaise, for serving

Sweet Barbecue Sauce (page 176),
   for serving

1 lime, quartered, for serving

1. In a food processor, combine the lentils and walnuts. Pulse 8 to 10 times until chopped. Make sure you don't process it into a purée. Leave chunks for a texture similar to ground beef. Transfer to a bowl.

2. Mix in the oil, cumin, oregano, chili powder, and salt. Taste, and adjust the seasoning, if desired.

3. Divide the bell pepper, scallions, cilantro, and cheese (if using) among 4 serving bowls.

4. Separate the lettuce leaves, and place on a platter. Top them with the walnut meat, mayonnaise, barbecue sauce, and lime juice.

FODMAP TIP: Watch for high-FODMAP ingredients such as garlic, onion, and inulin or chicory root in the vegan mayonnaise and vegan cheese.

Per Serving: Calories: 364; Total Fat: 26g; Saturated Fat: 3g; Cholesterol: 0mg; Sodium: 307mg; Carbohydrates: 26g; Fiber: 10g; Protein: 13g

Forbidden Edamame Bowl

VEGAN • 30 MINUTES OR LESS • MAKE AHEAD • ONE POT

SERVES 4 / PREP TIME: 15 MINUTES / COOK TIME: 15 MINUTES

It is a common misconception that edamame is forbidden on the low-FODMAP diet, but it's not true. You can enjoy edamame on the low-FODMAP diet (see the FODMAP Tip below). This colorful bowl makes a beautiful lunch or dinner. Edamame is an excellent source of protein, calcium, iron, omega-3 fats, and prebiotic fibers. Combined with quinoa and vegetables, this salad is a real powerhouse of nutrition.

1 cup quinoa

2 cups shelled edamame

1 carrot, shredded

1 red bell pepper, finely chopped

½ cup red cabbage, finely chopped

¼ cup chopped scallions, green parts only

½ to ¾ cup Goddess Dressing (page 179)

1. In a pot, prepare the quinoa according to the package instructions.
2. In a microwave-safe bowl, cook the edamame with 1 cup of water, uncovered, in the microwave for 3 to 5 minutes, or until tender.
3. In a large serving bowl, combine the quinoa and edamame. Place in the refrigerator for 5 minutes, or until cooled. Remove from the refrigerator.
4. Add the carrot, bell pepper, cabbage, and scallions, and gently mix.
5. Pour in the dressing, and combine well.

INGREDIENT TIP: Buy shelled edamame so you don't have to do it yourself.

COOKING TIP: Prepare the quinoa in advance so you can eliminate the cooling time when you make this recipe.

FODMAP TIP: A low-FODMAP serving is one-quarter of the recipe.

Per Serving: Calories: 335; Total Fat: 10g; Saturated Fat: 2g; Cholesterol: 0mg; Sodium: 425mg; Carbohydrates: 43g; Fiber: 8g; Protein: 19g

Vegan Rosé Spaghetti

VEGAN · 30 MINUTES OR LESS · MAKE AHEAD

SERVES 4 / PREP TIME: 10 MINUTES / COOK TIME: 20 MINUTES

Audrey would not be exaggerating when she says she's made this recipe more than 50 times for her family, with as many variations. But walnuts and basil are always a must in this recipe. The walnuts make it more like a creamy rosé than a traditional Bolognese. This pasta pairs nicely with steamed carrots, red bell peppers, or a mixed green salad. We recommend quinoa pasta to bump up your protein. Serve with a dollop of The Perfect Pesto (page 180).

12 ounces low-FODMAP pasta

2 tablespoons extra-virgin olive oil

1 red bell pepper, chopped

½ cup walnut pieces

1 (15-ounce) can diced tomatoes

2 tablespoons vegan red wine (optional)

¼ cup pitted, chopped Kalamata olives

1 cup chopped packed spinach leaves

Pinch salt

¼ cup chopped fresh basil leaves

Nutritional yeast, for serving (optional)

1. In a large pot, prepare the pasta according to the package instructions.
2. In a medium pot, heat the olive oil over medium-high heat.
3. Add the bell pepper, and sauté for 7 minutes, or until soft.
4. In a blender, process the walnuts until they are the texture of coarse sand.
5. To the pot with the bell pepper, add the walnuts, diced tomatoes and their juices, wine (if using), and olives. Stir to combine, and simmer for 20 minutes.
6. Add the spinach, stirring until wilted. Season with salt, and serve the sauce over the low-FODMAP pasta.
7. Garnish with the basil and nutritional yeast (if using).

VARIATION TIP: If you prefer, you can replace the walnuts with 1½ cups canned lentils.

COOKING TIP: To save time, use pitted and chopped olives. Keep a bag of spinach in your freezer, and add to sauces and stews to boost your iron intake.

Per Serving: Calories: 506; Total Fat: 18g; Saturated Fat: 2g; Cholesterol: 0mg; Sodium: 129mg; Carbohydrates: 73g; Fiber: 7g; Protein: 15g

Mediterranean Chickpeas

VEGAN · GLUTEN-FREE · 30 MINUTES OR LESS · MAKE AHEAD · ONE POT

SERVES 4 / PREP TIME: 15 MINUTES / COOK TIME: 15 MINUTES

We can't rave enough about chickpeas. They are a rich source of nutrition, containing protein, calcium, iron, and magnesium. Chickpeas are also loved by our gut bacteria as they provide a rich source of prebiotic fiber. We just have to make sure not to overindulge, as a larger serving will become high-FODMAP. This dish pairs nicely with rice or quinoa and a side salad.

1 tablespoon extra-virgin olive oil

1 cup chopped leeks, green parts only

1 teaspoon ground coriander

1 teaspoon ground cumin

Pinch salt

1 (15-ounce) can diced tomatoes

1 cup canned chickpeas, drained
    and rinsed

15 Kalamata olives, pitted and chopped

2 packed cups spinach, chopped

Grated zest and juice of 1 lemon

¼ cup chopped fresh basil (optional)

¼ cup chopped scallions, green
    parts only

Freshly ground black pepper

1. In a large pot, heat the oil over medium heat.
2. Add the leeks, coriander, cumin, and salt, and cook for 5 minutes, or until the leeks are soft.
3. Add the diced tomatoes and their juices, chickpeas, and olives. Reduce the heat to low, and simmer for 15 minutes, or until the flavors blend and the sauce has thickened. Remove from the heat.
4. Add the spinach and lemon zest and juice.
5. Divide among 4 bowls, and top with the basil (if using) and scallions. Season with pepper.

VARIATION TIP: Nonvegans can sprinkle ½ cup crumbled feta cheese over the 4 bowls for some extra tang.

COOKING TIP: This dish freezes well. Make a double batch, and save it for another week.

Per Serving: Calories: 156; Total Fat: 7g; Saturated Fat: 1g; Cholesterol: 0mg; Sodium: 170mg; Carbohydrates: 21g; Fiber: 6g; Protein: 6g

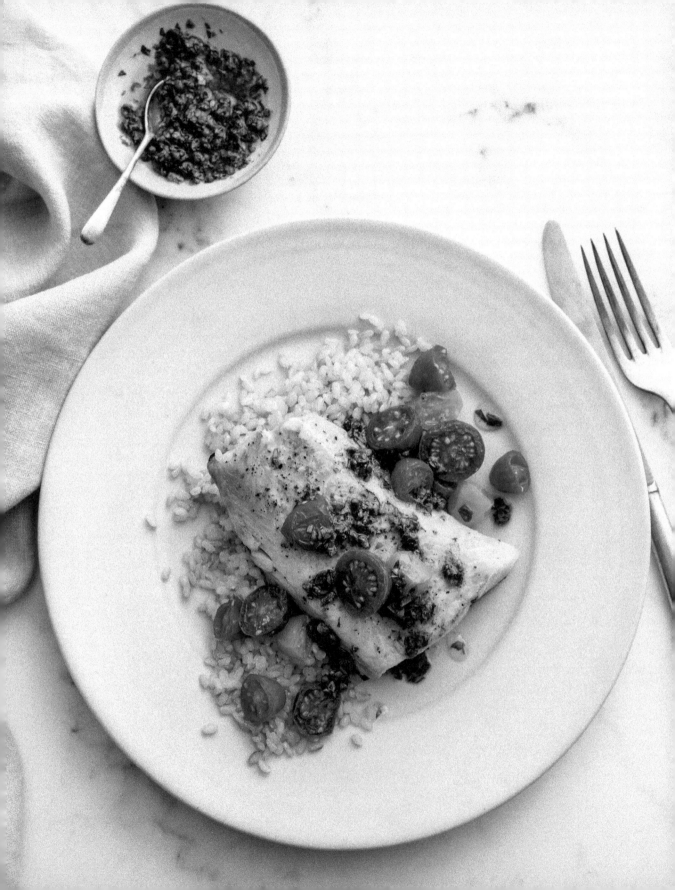

CHAPTER SEVEN

Fish and Seafood

Salmon with Basil-Caper Pesto, page 134

Maple-Mustard Rainbow Trout

GLUTEN-FREE • 30 MINUTES OR LESS • ONE POT

SERVES 4 / PREP TIME: 10 MINUTES / COOK TIME: 10 MINUTES

It has a crowd-pleasing mix of flavors, including sweet, savory, and a bit of spice from the ginger and pepper.

3 tablespoons extra-virgin olive oil

3 tablespoons maple syrup

3 tablespoons Dijon mustard

2 teaspoons freshly ground black pepper

1 teaspoon grated peeled fresh
   ginger (optional)

Nonstick cooking spray

1 pound fresh rainbow trout fillets
   or salmon

1. To make the sauce, in a small bowl, mix together the oil, maple syrup, mustard, pepper, and ginger (if using). Let sit for at least 10 minutes, or ideally for up to 2 hours, to let the flavors combine.

2. Preheat the oven to 400°F. Line a sheet pan with aluminum foil. Lightly grease the foil with cooking spray.

3. Place the fillets on the prepared sheet pan. Spoon the sauce over the fillets as evenly as possible.

4. Measure the fillets' thickness at the thickest point. Transfer the sheet pan to the oven, and bake for 10 minutes per inch of thickness. The fillets are done when they flake easily and the center of the thickest part has just turned an opaque pink. If the center is still a bright translucent pink, cook for another couple minutes or until opaque. Remove from the oven.

5. Store the leftovers in an airtight container in the refrigerator as soon as they have cooled off. Store for up to 4 days.

FODMAP TIP: Make sure to use Dijon mustard and not honey mustard, as honey becomes high-FODMAP in larger servings.

Per Serving: Calories: 283; Total Fat: 17g; Saturated Fat: 2g; Cholesterol: 0mg; Sodium: 135mg; Carbohydrates: 11g; Fiber: 1g; Protein: 23g

Canadian Maple Salmon

5 INGREDIENTS OR LESS • 30 MINUTES OR LESS • ONE POT

SERVES 2 / PREP TIME: 10 MINUTES / COOK TIME: 12 MINUTES

This recipe is melt-in-your-mouth delicious. We love salmon, as it is a rich source of omega-3 fats, which are great for heart health. Serve this dish with brown rice and a Caesar Salad (page 98), Kale Salad (page 94), or steamed green beans.

2 tablespoons soy sauce

2 tablespoons maple syrup

2 (6-ounce) salmon fillets

1. Preheat the oven to 400°F. Line a sheet pan with parchment paper.
2. In a medium bowl, combine the soy sauce and maple syrup.
3. Add the salmon, flesh-side down, to marinate for 10 minutes.
4. Place the salmon fillets on the prepared sheet pan, skin-side down. Cover with the sauce.
5. Transfer the sheet pan to the oven, and bake for 10 to 12 minutes, or until it is no longer opaque inside. Be careful not to overcook.

INGREDIENT TIP: Select fresh or frozen salmon fillets.

VARIATION TIP: Use 2 tablespoons brown sugar plus 2 tablespoons water instead of maple syrup.

Per Serving: Calories: 268; Total Fat: 6g; Saturated Fat: 2g; Cholesterol: 128mg; Sodium: 991mg; Carbohydrates: 15g; Fiber: 0g; Protein: 36g

Tuna Melt

30 MINUTES OR LESS • ONE POT

SERVES 2 / PREP TIME: 5 MINUTES / COOK TIME: 5 MINUTES

This open-face tuna melt is a great sandwich that works for both lunch and dinner. It pairs nicely with the Carrot-Ginger Soup (page 90), Caesar Salad (page 98), or cut vegetables like cucumber, carrots, and red bell peppers.

2 (6-ounce) cans water-packed
  tuna, drained

¼ cup mayonnaise

¼ cup chopped scallions, green
  parts only

2 dill pickles (no garlic), finely
  chopped (optional)

4 low-FODMAP bread slices, toasted

1 cup shredded mozzarella cheese

1. Set the oven to broil.
2. In a medium bowl, mix together the tuna, mayonnaise, scallions, and pickles (if using).
3. Place the pieces of toast on a sheet pan. Divide the tuna mixture between the pieces of toast, and top with the cheese.
4. Transfer the sheet pan to the top rack of the oven, and broil for 2 to 3 minutes, or until the cheese is melted and bubbly.

COOKING TIP: Instead of melting the cheese in the oven, you can place the tuna melts in the microwave two at a time for about 30 seconds, or until the cheese is melted.

VARIATION TIP: Instead of mozzarella, use Cheddar. Instead of tuna, try it with salmon or chicken.

Per Serving: Calories: 685; Total Fat: 39g; Saturated Fat: 13g; Cholesterol: 102mg; Sodium: 512mg; Carbohydrates: 26g; Fiber: 4g; Protein: 57g

Tuna Pasta

30 MINUTES OR LESS • ONE POT

SERVES 4 / PREP TIME: 10 MINUTES / COOK TIME: 15 MINUTES

This tuna pasta is the perfect answer to what to eat for dinner at the end of the grocery week. It can be entirely pulled together in minutes with items from your pantry. Serve it with the Pomegranate, Poppy Seed, and Spinach Salad (page 102), sliced raw vegetables (carrots, red peppers, cucumbers), or steamed carrots.

12 ounces low-FODMAP pasta

2 (6-ounce) cans water-packed tuna, drained

½ cup chopped pitted Kalamata olives

¼ cup chopped fresh basil leaves or 1 tablespoon dried basil leaves

2 tablespoons extra-virgin olive oil

2 tablespoons finely chopped sun-dried tomatoes (optional)

½ cup grated Parmesan cheese

1. Bring a large pot of water to a boil over high heat, and prepare the pasta according to the package instructions.

2. In a medium bowl, use a fork to combine the tuna, olives, basil, oil, and sun-dried tomatoes (if using). Break the tuna apart into smaller pieces, and mix well.

3. Divide the pasta and the tuna mixture among 4 bowls.

4. Top with the cheese.

COOKING TIP: Buy pitted Kalamata olives to save prep time.

VARIATION TIP: Try green olives or capers instead of Kalamatas.

Per Serving: Calories: 613; Total Fat: 15g; Saturated Fat: 4g; Cholesterol: 95mg; Sodium: 523mg; Carbohydrates: 65g; Fiber: 3g; Protein: 53g

Salmon with Basil-Caper Pesto

GLUTEN-FREE · 5 INGREDIENTS OR LESS · 30 MINUTES OR LESS · ONE POT

SERVES 2 / PREP TIME: 5 MINUTES / COOK TIME: 10 MINUTES

Here's a variation on your usual salmon fillet. It is served with a fresh basil-caper pesto and cherry tomatoes, which make for quite a flavor combination. Serve it with a simple mixed green salad with Maple–Balsamic Vinegar Dressing (page 181) and rice or quinoa.

3 tablespoons extra-virgin olive oil, divided

2 (4- to 6-ounce) salmon fillets

1½ cups halved cherry tomatoes

Pinch salt

Freshly ground black pepper

¼ cup basil leaves or 2 tablespoons dried basil

2 tablespoons capers

1. In a large skillet, heat 1 tablespoon of oil over medium heat.
2. Add the salmon, skin-side down, and tomatoes, then season with the salt and pepper. Cook for 3 to 4 minutes, then flip the salmon and cook the other side for 3 to 4 minutes, or until the fish is cooked through and no longer translucent in the thickest part.
3. Mince the basil and capers together to encourage them to blend. Transfer to a small bowl, and add the remaining 2 tablespoons of oil. Stir well, and mash with a fork to combine.
4. Divide the salmon, tomatoes, and basil-caper mixture between 2 plates, and serve.

VARIATION TIP: Instead of capers, use black or green olives. Instead of basil, try parsley.

Per Serving: Calories: 408; Total Fat: 33g; Saturated Fat: 6g; Cholesterol: 65mg; Sodium: 304mg; Carbohydrates: 6g; Fiber: 2g; Protein: 24g

Ginger-Lime Salmon Burgers

30 MINUTES OR LESS · MAKE AHEAD · ONE POT

SERVES 4 / PREP TIME: 10 MINUTES / COOK TIME: 10 MINUTES

Here's an Asian variation of your usual salmon burger. Enjoy it on a gluten-free bun with a few leaves of spinach, a slice of tomato, and one of the dips in our Creamy Dipping Duo (page 182). You can also eat it wrapped in a leaf of butter lettuce. These salmon burgers go well with a mixed green salad and Goddess Dressing (page 179).

2 (6-ounce) cans salmon, drained

1 large egg, beaten

½ cup finely chopped scallions, green parts only

⅓ cup gluten-free bread crumbs

Grated zest and juice of ½ lime

1 tablespoon grated peeled fresh ginger

1 teaspoon extra-virgin olive oil

4 low-FODMAP hamburger buns

1 tomato, thinly sliced

1 cup baby spinach leaves

1. In a medium bowl, combine the salmon, egg, scallions, bread crumbs, lime zest and juice, and ginger. Stir with a fork until the mixture is thoroughly incorporated, then finish mixing it with your hands.

2. Shape ½-cup portions of the mixture into 4 (1-inch-thick) patties.

3. In a large skillet, heat the oil over medium-high heat.

4. Add the patties, and cook, flipping once, for 4 to 5 minutes on each side, or until crispy and golden brown. Serve on buns topped with tomato and spinach.

COOKING TIP: Freeze the leftover cooked burgers to enjoy on another day. They will keep in the freezer for 3 months.

FODMAP TIP: Enjoy your burger with condiments like mayonnaise and mustard. If you choose ketchup, limit it to 1 teaspoon, as ketchup can become high-FODMAP with a larger amount.

Per Serving: Calories: 233; Total Fat: 8g; Saturated Fat: 2g; Cholesterol: 75mg; Sodium: 387mg; Carbohydrates: 24g; Fiber: 6g; Protein: 22g

Buttered Shrimp with Fresh Cilantro

GLUTEN-FREE • 5 INGREDIENTS OR LESS • 30 MINUTES OR LESS • ONE POT

SERVES 4 / PREP TIME: 2 MINUTES / COOK TIME: 10 MINUTES

These succulent shrimp go well with just about anything. You will definitely appreciate the Garlic-Infused Oil and butter combination. Add these shrimp to one of our salads, or have them with the Sweet Potato Quinoa Cakes (page 97).

2 tablespoons butter

2 tablespoons Garlic-Infused Oil (page 184) or extra-virgin olive oil

1 pound peeled, deveined shrimp

½ cup chopped fresh cilantro

¼ cup freshly squeezed lime juice

Freshly ground black pepper

1. In a large skillet, melt the butter over medium heat.
2. Add the oil and shrimp. Cook, flipping once halfway through, for 4 to 5 minutes, or until the shrimp is pink on both sides.
3. Add the cilantro and lime juice. Cook for 2 to 3 minutes, or until the flavors meld. Season with pepper.

INGREDIENT TIP: Buy shrimp that are already deveined and shelled to save time.

VARIATION TIP: Try with white wine instead of lime juice. If you're not a cilantro fan, fresh basil, fresh parsley, or dried Italian seasoning are equally delicious.

Per Serving: Calories: 212; Total Fat: 14g; Saturated Fat: 5g; Cholesterol: 195mg; Sodium: 171mg; Carbohydrates: 0g; Fiber: 0g; Protein: 23g

Shrimp Fettuccine

GLUTEN-FREE • 30 MINUTES OR LESS

SERVES 4 / PREP TIME: 10 MINUTES / COOK TIME: 20 MINUTES

This is the shrimp fettuccine that you probably thought you couldn't have. Our version is made low-FODMAP just for you. Serve it with steamed green beans or a mixed green salad.

12 ounces low-FODMAP fettuccine

1 teaspoon extra-virgin olive oil

1 pound shrimp, peeled and deveined

Freshly ground black pepper

2 tablespoons butter

1 small zucchini, very thinly sliced

Pinch salt

1 cup lactose-free half-and-half

½ cup grated Parmesan cheese

1 lemon, cut into wedges, for garnish

1 tablespoon chopped parsley,
   for garnish

1. Bring a large pot of water to a boil over high heat, and prepare the pasta according to the package instructions.

2. In a large skillet, heat the oil over medium heat.

3. Add the shrimp, and season with pepper. Cook for 4 to 5 minutes, flipping once halfway through, or until they turn pink. Transfer to a bowl.

4. In the same skillet, melt the butter over medium-high heat.

5. Add the zucchini. Season with the salt and pepper. Cook for 5 minutes, or until translucent. Remove from the heat, and let cool for 5 minutes.

6. Slowly add the half-and-half and cheese to the same skillet while stirring. Simmer over low heat for 2 minutes, or until the cheese has melted.

7. Add the pasta and shrimp. Toss to coat. Serve with lemon wedges, and garnish with parsley.

COOKING TIP: Buy shrimp that is already peeled and deveined. Don't underestimate how quickly shrimp cooks. Small shrimp can literally be done in 2 minutes.

VARIATION TIP: Use pre-grated Parmesan to save time on grating.

Per Serving: Calories: 527; Total Fat: 29g; Saturated Fat: 8g; Cholesterol: 315mg; Sodium: 523mg; Carbohydrates: 36g; Fiber: 5g; Protein: 39g

Lemon-Pepper Pickerel

GLUTEN-FREE • 5 INGREDIENTS OR LESS • 30 MINUTES OR LESS • ONE POT

SERVES 4 / PREP TIME: 10 MINUTES / COOK TIME: 5 MINUTES

Most summers, Lauren visits northern Ontario, where she has the opportunity to go fishing with her family and catch pickerel (walleye). This recipe is from her dad's best friend Hannu, and it tastes best with the freshest whitefish you can find (or catch!). Our friend Joyce said this recipe long ago converted her to eating fish. The key is to not get too much flour on the fish; aim for a nice even coating. We doubt there will be any leftovers, but if there are, don't reheat the fish. Eat it cold within a few days.

1 pound pickerel fillets or other whitefish

1½ teaspoons lemon-pepper seasoning

2 tablespoons low-FODMAP all-purpose flour

1 tablespoon canola oil

1 teaspoon butter

4 lemon slices (optional)

1. Rinse the fillets with cold water. On both sides, sprinkle with lemon-pepper seasoning, then lightly, evenly coat with flour.

2. In a medium skillet, heat the oil over medium-high heat, and add the butter.

3. Once the butter has melted and the oil is hot and sizzling (be careful not to burn), add the fillets. Cook for 2 to 3 minutes, or until the outside of the fillets has turned white or opaque and the bottom has lightly browned.

4. Flip the fillets, and cook for 2 minutes, or until the fillets flake easily and both sides have browned.

5. Serve with lemon slices (if using). Store leftovers in an airtight container in the refrigerator for up to 4 days.

COOKING TIP: This cooks fast! Keep your eye on it, and avoid overcooking. The cooking time will vary slightly based on the temperature of the oil. As soon as the fish is opaque and flakes easily at the thickest part, remove from the heat.

VARIATION TIP: You can use any whitefish you prefer. Try tilapia or sole; both are mild-tasting options.

FODMAP TIP: Read the ingredient list of lemon-pepper seasonings carefully and avoid brands with garlic or onion.

Per Serving: Calories: 203; Total Fat: 10g; Saturated Fat: 1g; Cholesterol: 3mg; Sodium: 12mg; Carbohydrates: 3g; Fiber: 0g; Protein: 23g

Fish in a Bag

GLUTEN-FREE · 30 MINUTES OR LESS · ONE POT

SERVES 4 / PREP TIME: 10 MINUTES / COOK TIME: 10 TO 20 MINUTES

It's easy to make a bag using parchment paper and staples. Cooking the fish, vegetables, and oil together in the bag seals in the flavor. You can vary this recipe by using different types of fish, vegetables, and seasonings. It's nice to serve on top of brown rice or quinoa.

1 pound tilapia fillets (or other neutral whitefish)

1½ tablespoons Cajun Spice Mix (page 186), divided

1 red bell pepper, chopped

½ cup chopped broccoli

½ cup chopped zucchini

1 tablespoon Onion-Infused Oil (page 185), Garlic-Infused Oil (page 184), or extra-virgin olive oil

1. Preheat the oven to 400°F. Cut a piece of parchment paper approximately 1½ times the size of your sheet pan. Place the parchment paper on the sheet pan.

2. Place the fillets on the parchment paper. Season with ¾ tablespoon of Cajun Spice Mix.

3. Cover the fillets with the bell pepper, broccoli, and zucchini. Drizzle with the Onion-Infused Oil, and season with the remaining ¾ tablespoon of spice mix.

4. Measure the fillets' thickness at the thickest point. Fold the parchment paper over, and make a "bag" by folding the ends up, then stapling to seal it shut.

5. Transfer the sheet pan to the oven, and bake for 10 minutes per inch of thickness. The fillets are done when they flake easily and have turned opaque (internal temperature should reach 158°F). Remove from the oven.

INGREDIENT TIP: Try to purchase fillets that have fairly even thickness, if possible. Make sure to measure the thickness of the fillets at the thickest part before placing the fish on the parchment paper.

VARIATION TIP: Instead of Cajun Spice Mix, try lemon-pepper seasoning or Italian seasoning, or any other low-FODMAP seasonings you love. Each family member can have their own bag with their own seasonings. Kids can have fun choosing what to put in their bag.

Per Serving: Calories: 139; Total Fat: 5g; Saturated Fat: 1g; Cholesterol: 55mg; Sodium: 46mg; Carbohydrates: 4g; Fiber: 1g; Protein: 22g

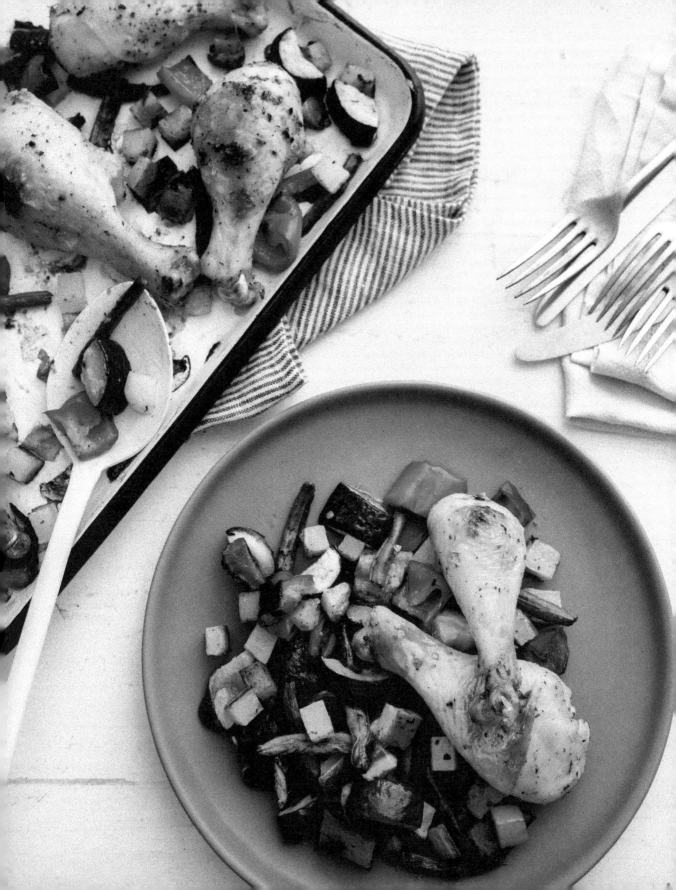

CHAPTER EIGHT

Poultry and Meat

Sheet Pan Chicken and Vegetables, page 148

Coconut Chicken Strips

30 MINUTES OR LESS • ONE POT

SERVES 4 / PREP TIME: 10 MINUTES / COOK TIME: 20 MINUTES

This is a tropical twist on classic chicken strips. The coconut breading gets nicely browned and crispy in the oven. On the side, try out the Warm Roasted Vegetable Salad (page 104) or Crispy Parmesan Baby Potatoes (page 101) with Pomegranate, Poppy Seed, and Spinach Salad (page 102). The Creamy Dipping Duo (page 182) is an absolute must!

Extra-virgin olive oil, for greasing

⅓ cup low-FODMAP flour blend

1 teaspoon dried basil

¼ teaspoon salt

⅛ teaspoon freshly ground black pepper

1 large egg

¾ cup shredded unsweetened
   dried coconut

¼ cup bread crumbs

1 pound boneless, skinless chicken
   breasts (2 large breasts), cut
   lengthwise into strips

1. Preheat the oven to 400°F. Lightly grease a sheet pan with oil, or cover it with parchment paper.

2. In a small bowl, mix together the flour, basil, salt, and pepper.

3. Crack the egg into another bowl, and beat.

4. In a third bowl, mix together the coconut and bread crumbs.

5. Lightly coat each chicken strip with the flour mixture, followed by the egg, then the coconut bread crumbs, and place onto the prepared sheet pan.

6. Transfer the sheet pan to the oven. Bake for 10 minutes, then carefully flip each chicken strip. Return to the oven, and bake for another 8 minutes, or until the coconut has browned and the chicken is cooked through. (The internal temperature should reach 165°F.) Remove from the oven. Store leftovers in the refrigerator for up to 4 days.

COOKING TIP: For this recipe, we typically cut large chicken breasts into 5 strips. Do your best to make them approximately the same thickness so they cook evenly. It's okay if they are varying in lengths.

INGREDIENT TIP: Make sure you buy unsweetened shredded coconut, not the sweetened version.

Per Serving: Calories: 369; Total Fat: 19g; Saturated Fat: 14g; Cholesterol: 112mg; Sodium: 275mg; Carbohydrates: 16g; Fiber: 4g; Protein: 31g

Chive-Rubbed Chicken

GLUTEN-FREE • 5 INGREDIENTS OR LESS •
30 MINUTES OR LESS • MAKE AHEAD • ONE POT

SERVES 2 / PREP TIME: 5 MINUTES / COOK TIME: 15 MINUTES

There's nothing easier than throwing a juicy piece of chicken on the grill for dinner. This chicken is designed to blend into any meal. It is the perfect way to turn any of our yummy salads, like Caesar Salad (page 98), Greek Quinoa Salad (page 96), or Cranberry-Quinoa Salad (page 100) into a complete meal.

1 (8-ounce) boneless, skinless
   chicken breast

2 tablespoons dried chives or minced
   scallions, green parts only

Pinch salt

Freshly ground black pepper

1 teaspoon extra-virgin olive
   oil (optional)

1. Preheat a grill on medium heat.

2. Pound the chicken breast to about ½-inch thickness, and rub each side with the chives, salt, and pepper. Let sit for 5 minutes.

3. Place the chicken on the grates, and grill, flipping once, for 6 minutes per side, or until the juices run clear.

4. Alternatively, on the stove, in a large skillet, heat the oil (if using) over medium heat. Cook the chicken breast, flipping once, for 6 minutes per side, or until golden brown and cooked through.

5. Cut the chicken into bite-size pieces, and serve.

VARIATION TIP: Add cumin, Italian seasoning, dried oregano, or dried basil to the rub.

COOKING TIP: Pounding the chicken helps it cook faster and more evenly. Cook a few breasts and store them in the freezer for a quick and easy meal on another day.

INGREDIENT TIP: Choose boneless chicken thighs instead of breasts.

Per Serving: Calories: 131; Total Fat: 3g; Saturated Fat: 0g; Cholesterol: 73mg; Sodium: 136mg; Carbohydrates: 0g; Fiber: 0g; Protein: 24g

Sun-Dried Tomato and Feta Chicken Sliders

GLUTEN-FREE • 5 INGREDIENTS OR LESS • 30 MINUTES OR LESS • MAKE AHEAD • ONE POT

SERVES 4 [2 SLIDERS = 1 SERVING] / PREP TIME: 10 MINUTES / COOK TIME: 15 MINUTES

You will love the small bursts of rich feta as you sink your teeth into these patties. You can finish them with your favorite toppings like sliced tomato, lettuce, and mayonnaise. Enjoy on a low-FODMAP bun or wrapped in lettuce.

1 pound ground chicken

½ cup crumbled feta cheese

2 (1-ounce) sun-dried tomato pieces in oil, finely chopped

¼ cup chopped fresh basil

¼ cup chopped scallions, green parts only

¼ teaspoon salt (optional)

Freshly ground black pepper

1. In a medium bowl, combine the chicken, cheese, sun-dried tomatoes, basil, and scallions. Season with salt (if using) and pepper. Knead with your hands until uniform and well-mixed. Leave a few larger chunks of cheese.

2. Shape ¼-cup portions of the mixture into 8 (1-inch-thick) patties.

3. Heat a large nonstick skillet over medium-high heat.

4. Add the patties, and cook, flipping once, for 10 to 12 minutes, or until browned on each side and cooked through. Remove from the heat.

COOKING TIP: These sliders will keep in the freezer for up to 1 month.

Per Serving (2 sliders): Calories: 234; Total Fat: 15g; Saturated Fat: 5g; Cholesterol: 113mg; Sodium: 278mg; Carbohydrates: 2g; Fiber: 0g; Protein: 23g

Prosciutto-Wrapped Chicken

GLUTEN-FREE · 5 INGREDIENTS OR LESS · 30 MINUTES OR LESS · ONE POT

SERVES 4 / PREP TIME: 8 MINUTES / COOK TIME: 20 MINUTES

Imagine a lovely breast of chicken hugged by a crispy thin layer of prosciutto. A photo of this chicken is absolutely worthy of a magazine cover. Serve the chicken with steamed green beans and Crispy Parmesan Baby Potatoes (page 101) or with a Caprese Salad (page 93) and The Perfect Pesto (page 180) on the side.

1 pound boneless, skinless chicken breasts (2 large breasts), cut lengthwise in half

8 slices prosciutto (4 ounces)

1 tablespoon butter, melted

Fresh oregano sprigs or dried oregano leaves, for garnish

¼ cup The Perfect Pesto (page 180) (optional)

1. Preheat the oven to 450°F.
2. Wrap each piece of chicken with 2 slices of prosciutto. Press gently to adhere. Place on a sheet pan. Brush with the melted butter.
3. Transfer the sheet pan to the oven, and bake for 18 minutes, or until the chicken has cooked through. Remove from the oven.
4. Garnish the chicken with oregano, and serve with the pesto (if using).

COOKING TIP: Use a meat thermometer to check that the internal temperature is 165°F. Don't cut the chicken with a knife to check for doneness, as the juices will leak out and the chicken will be less moist.

Per Serving: Calories: 236; Total Fat: 9g; Saturated Fat: 3g; Cholesterol: 102mg; Sodium: 511mg; Carbohydrates: 1g; Fiber: 0g; Protein: 36g

Chicken Cacciatore

GLUTEN-FREE • MAKE AHEAD • ONE POT

SERVES 4 / PREP TIME: 10 MINUTES / COOK TIME: 35 MINUTES

Chicken Cacciatore is a classic Italian dish that will warm your belly and your kitchen on a cool day. Serve it on a bed of low-FODMAP pasta.

2 tablespoons Garlic-Infused Oil
   (page 184) or extra-virgin olive oil

1 cup chopped leeks, green parts only

1 carrot, peeled and chopped

1 red bell pepper, chopped

1¼ pounds bone-in chicken thighs
   (4 thighs)

2 cups canned crushed tomatoes

½ cup chopped pitted Kalamata olives

2 teaspoons dried oregano

Pinch salt

Freshly ground black pepper

1. In a large pot, heat the oil over medium-high heat.
2. Add the leeks, carrot, and bell pepper, and sauté for 7 minutes, or until soft.
3. Add the chicken thighs, and sauté, flipping once, for 5 minutes, or until seared on both sides.

4. Add the tomatoes, olives, and oregano, reduce the heat to low, and simmer for 20 minutes, or until the chicken has cooked through. Divide among 4 bowls. Season with the salt and pepper.

COOKING TIP: You can prepare this dish in advance and reheat it on the stovetop. It freezes really well and will keep for up to 3 months in the freezer.

INGREDIENT TIP: You can use any cut of chicken, such as breasts, thighs, or drumsticks.

VARIATION TIP: Add a splash of red wine if you have a bottle open.

Per Serving: Calories: 461; Total Fat: 30g; Saturated Fat: 8g; Cholesterol:119mg; Sodium: 457mg; Carbohydrates: 18g; Fiber: 6g; Protein: 29g

Orange Chicken and Broccoli Bowl

ONE POT

SERVES 4 / PREP TIME: 20 MINUTES / COOK TIME: 15 MINUTES

This dish will satisfy your fiercest craving for takeout. Have it with rice or quinoa on the days you need a little extra energy.

1 tablespoon sesame oil

1½ pounds chicken thighs, cut into bite-size pieces

½ cup Nourishing Vegetable Broth (page 178) or low-FODMAP chicken broth

Grated zest and juice of 1 orange

¼ cup brown sugar

¼ cup soy sauce

3 cups broccoli florets, cut into bite-size pieces

3 cups sliced peeled carrots

¼ cup chopped scallions, green parts only

2 tablespoons sesame seeds

1. In a large skillet, heat the oil over medium heat.

2. Add the chicken, and cook for 5 to 7 minutes, or until cooked through and browned. Remove from the heat.

3. In a small saucepan, stir together the broth, orange zest and juice, sugar, and soy sauce. Bring to a boil, then reduce the heat to a simmer, and cook for 8 to 10 minutes, or until thickened slightly.

4. Pour the mixture over the chicken in the skillet. Mix well to coat.

5. In a medium pot, combine the broccoli, carrots, and about ½ cup water. Place over medium-high heat, and cook for 5 minutes, or until tender. Divide among 4 bowls, and top with the chicken, scallions, and sesame seeds.

COOKING TIP: To save time, use baby carrots and a bag of prewashed broccoli heads.

FODMAP TIP: Trim off and discard the broccoli stems; use mostly broccoli heads, as the stems are higher in FODMAPs.

Per Serving: Calories: 395; Total Fat: 13g; Saturated Fat: 2g; Cholesterol: 143mg; Sodium: 1053mg; Carbohydrates: 33g; Fiber: 6g; Protein: 37g

Sheet Pan Chicken and Vegetables

GLUTEN-FREE • ONE POT

SERVES 4 / PREP TIME: 10 MINUTES / COOK TIME: 25 MINUTES

Sheet pan dinners are a new discovery for Audrey. The selling features are that they take only a few minutes to prepare and there's only one pan to clean afterward. So nice. Sheet pan meals are a great way to squeeze in loads of delicious low-FODMAP vegetables, too.

2 tablespoons extra-virgin olive oil

1 tablespoon Italian seasoning

4 to 6 chicken drumsticks

2 medium potatoes, cut into ½-inch dice

1 cup coarsely chopped zucchini

1 red bell pepper, cut into 1-inch pieces

1 cup cut (1-inch) green beans

Pinch salt

Freshly ground black pepper

1. Preheat the oven to 400°F.
2. In a large bowl, combine the oil and Italian seasoning, and mix well.
3. Add the chicken, potatoes, zucchini, bell pepper, and green beans. Mix gently to coat. Season with the salt and pepper. Place on a sheet pan.
4. Transfer the sheet pan to the oven, and cook for 25 minutes, or until the chicken has cooked through and the vegetables are tender. Remove from the oven. Divide among 4 plates, and serve.

COOKING TIP: Cut the zucchini, peppers, and green beans to a similar size so they take the same length of time to cook. Cut the potatoes smaller.

VARIATION TIP: Try this dish with the Cajun Spice Mix (page 186) instead of the Italian seasoning. Use carrots and parsnips instead of zucchini and green beans.

Per Serving: Calories: 377; Total Fat: 22g; Saturated Fat: 5g; Cholesterol: 97mg; Sodium: 142mg; Carbohydrates: 22g; Fiber: 4g; Protein: 24g

Turkey Burgers

30 MINUTES OR LESS • ONE POT

SERVES 4 / PREP TIME: 5 MINUTES / COOK TIME: 15 MINUTES

Turkey burgers are a healthy, lower-fat alternative to beef burgers. It's much easier to make them yourself than trying to find a premade low-FODMAP burger in stores. It can be challenging to find buns that are low-FODMAP and taste good. Lauren often prefers to serve her burger on a bed of greens or between slices of sourdough bread. Serve with the Creamy Dipping Duo (page 182).

1 pound ground turkey

1 large egg

¼ cup rolled oats

1 tablespoon Worcestershire sauce

½ teaspoon freshly ground black pepper

¼ teaspoon salt

1. Preheat a grill on medium heat.
2. In a large bowl, mix together the turkey, egg, oats, Worcestershire sauce, pepper, and salt. Shape into 4 patties that are about 4 inches wide and ¾ inch thick.
3. Place the patties on the grates, and grill for about 6 minutes, or until the bottoms have grill marks.
4. Flip the patties, and cook for 3 to 5 minutes, or until the juices run clear and the inside is no longer pink. (The temperature of the burgers should reach 165°F at the thickest part.)

5. Divide the burgers among 4 plates. Store leftovers in the refrigerator for up to 4 days.

SUBSTITUTION TIP: Low-FODMAP bread crumbs can be used instead of rolled oats.

COOKING TIP: You can make these on a stove instead of on a grill. Use a large greased skillet over medium heat.

Per Serving: Calories: 167; Total Fat: 4g; Saturated Fat: 1g; Cholesterol: 109mg; Sodium: 263mg; Carbohydrates: 5g; Fiber: 1g; Protein: 29g

Pork Tenderloin Medallions

5 INGREDIENTS OR LESS · ONE POT

SERVES 4 / PREP TIME: 4 HOURS / COOK TIME: 10 MINUTES

Our orange-ginger marinade helps make this pork tenderloin extra juicy. Tenderloin is a lean cut of meat, but be sure to slice off any visible fat to help prevent flare-ups on the grill. You can grill this for added flavor, or you can roast it in the oven. If you are grilling, we suggest serving the pork with grilled pineapple slices.

1 pound pork tenderloin, trimmed of fat, cut into ¾-inch-thick medallions

¾ cup Orange-Ginger Marinade (page 189)

1. In a storage container or bowl, combine the pork and marinade, and refrigerate for at least 4 hours.
2. Preheat a grill on medium-high heat to about 450°F.
3. Place the pork on the grates, and grill, flipping once, for 4 minutes per side. The pork is done when there are grill marks on both sides, there is no dark pink in middle (light pink is okay), and the internal temperature reaches 145°F. Remove from the heat, and let rest for 5 minutes before serving. Store in the refrigerator for up to 4 days.

COOKING TIP: Instead of grilling, you can roast the pork on a sheet pan in a 450°F oven for the same amount of time, flipping once about halfway through.

INGREDIENT TIP: Carefully slice the pork so the thickness is a maximum of ¾ inch.

Per Serving: Calories: 175; Total Fat: 9g; Saturated Fat: 3g; Cholesterol: 65mg; Sodium: 797mg; Carbohydrates: 3g; Fiber: 0g; Protein: 21g

Barbecue Pulled Pork

GLUTEN-FREE • 5 INGREDIENTS OR LESS • MAKE AHEAD • ONE POT

SERVES 4 / PREP TIME: 10 MINUTES / COOK TIME: 9 HOURS

There are multiple ways to cook pulled pork, depending on what you have available. You can do it in the slow cooker, Instant Pot®, or oven. Pulled pork is best enjoyed on a low-FODMAP bun with Classic Coleslaw with a Lime Twist (page 95).

1 pound pork tenderloin

1 recipe Sweet Barbecue Sauce (page 176)

TO MAKE IN THE SLOW COOKER

1. Cut the pork in half widthwise.
2. In a slow cooker, combine the pork with the barbecue sauce. Cover, and set on low for 9 hours.
3. Carefully remove the lid and, using 2 forks, shred the pork.

TO MAKE IN THE INSTANT POT®

1. Cut the pork in half widthwise.
2. Set the Instant Pot® on Sauté, and sear the pork on all sides until browned.
3. Add the barbecue sauce, and turn to coat.
4. Close and lock the lid, and pressure-cook on high for 45 minutes. Once cooking is complete, naturally release the pressure.
5. Carefully remove the lid and, using 2 forks, shred the pork.

COOKING TIP: The pork should fall apart easily. If it is difficult to pull apart, it may need additional cooking time. This is a perfect recipe for batch cooking. Marinate the pork in the barbecue sauce, and store in the freezer for up to 4 months. Defrost in the refrigerator overnight, and place in the slow cooker the next morning.

Per Serving: Calories: 212; Total Fat: 4g; Saturated Fat: 2g; Cholesterol: 65mg; Sodium: 428mg; Carbohydrates: 22g; Fiber: 2g; Protein: 22g

Sheet Pan Steak and Potatoes

GLUTEN-FREE • ONE POT

SERVES 4 / PREP TIME: 10 MINUTES / COOK TIME: 25 MINUTES

Although beef is sometimes treated harshly during production, we like it because it is an excellent source of highly absorbable iron, which is great to prevent and treat iron-deficiency anemia. And sheet pan dinners like this one are really fast and delicious.

4 cups diced (½-inch) potatoes

3 red bell peppers, cut into 1-inch dice

1 tablespoon extra-virgin olive oil

½ teaspoon salt, divided

Freshly ground black pepper

1 pound rib eye steak, cut into
**   1-inch dice**

⅓ cup chopped scallions, green
**   parts only**

1. Preheat the oven to 400°F. Line a sheet pan with parchment paper.

2. In a large bowl, combine the potatoes, peppers, oil, and ¼ teaspoon of salt. Season with pepper, and mix well. Transfer to the prepared sheet pan.

3. Transfer the sheet pan to the oven, and cook for 10 minutes.

4. Season the steak with the remaining ¼ teaspoon of salt and pepper.

5. Remove the sheet pan from the oven, and carefully stir in the beef. Return to the oven, and bake for 15 minutes, or until the beef is cooked to your desired level of doneness. Garnish with scallions.

VARIATION TIP: You can use a different type of grilling beef, pork, or chicken.

Per Serving: Calories: 405; Total Fat: 16g; Saturated Fat: 5g; Cholesterol: 100mg; Sodium: 401mg; Carbohydrates: 31g; Fiber: 5g; Protein: 34g

Chile-Lime DIY Tacos

GLUTEN-FREE

SERVES 4 / PREP TIME: 20 MINUTES / COOK TIME: 15 MINUTES

This is a meal that will make everyone at the dinner table happy because they build their own tacos. Tacos go well with a bag of coleslaw or cut vegetables like cucumber and red pepper. As dietitians, we love to extend ground beef with black beans to add prebiotic fiber, antioxidants, protein, and iron.

8 ounces lean ground beef

1 cup canned black beans, drained and rinsed

¼ cup water

2 tablespoons ancho chile powder (no garlic)

Pinch salt (optional)

½ lettuce head, any type, chopped

1 cup Fresh Cut Salsa (page 177)

½ cup shredded Cheddar cheese

½ cup lactose-free sour cream

⅓ cup finely chopped scallions, green parts only

4 large or 8 small corn tortillas

1 lime, quartered

1. In a large skillet, cook the ground beef over medium-high heat for 8 minutes, or until it is no longer pink. Break up the large pieces into smaller pieces. Carefully drain off and discard any fat.

2. Add the beans, water, chile powder, and salt (if using). Mash some of the beans with a wooden spoon to create a saucy mixture. Transfer to a serving bowl.

3. Divide the lettuce, salsa, cheese, sour cream, and scallions among individual serving bowls.

4. Place a clean pan over high heat. When hot, heat the tortillas one at a time, 20 to 30 seconds per side, and keep warm wrapped in a clean kitchen towel.

5. Everyone can make their own tacos by placing ¼ of the beef and bean mixture in a tortilla and topping it with lettuce, salsa, cheese, sour cream, and scallions. Garnish with lime.

VARIATION TIP: You can use 1 cup canned lentils instead of black beans.

Per Serving: Calories: 403; Total Fat: 17g; Saturated Fat: 13g; Cholesterol: 62mg; Sodium: 377mg; Carbohydrates: 45g; Fiber: 9g; Protein: 23g

Spaghetti Bolognese

GLUTEN-FREE

SERVES 4 / PREP TIME: 10 MINUTES / COOK TIME: 30 MINUTES

Everyone needs a delicious and quick Bolognese. Audrey could serve this every day and her family would never complain. Enjoy it with a Caesar Salad (page 98), steamed carrots, or steamed green beans.

12 ounces low-FODMAP spaghetti

1 pound lean ground beef

1 tablespoon extra-virgin olive oil

1 cup chopped leeks, green parts only

1 red bell pepper, chopped

2 cups tomato sauce or passata

2 teaspoons Italian seasoning

1 cup chopped spinach

½ cup grated Parmesan cheese

1. Bring a large pot of water to a boil over high heat, and prepare the spaghetti according to the package instructions.

2. In a large pot, cook the ground beef over medium-high heat for 10 minutes, or until it is no longer pink. Break it up into smaller pieces. Carefully drain off and discard any fat, and transfer the beef to a bowl.

3. In the same pot, heat the oil over medium-high heat.

4. Add the leeks and bell pepper, and sauté for 8 minutes, or until soft.

5. Add the tomato sauce, beef, and Italian seasoning. Simmer for 10 minutes, or until the flavors meld.

6. Add the spinach and cheese, and mix well.

7. Divide the spaghetti among 4 plates, and top with the sauce.

COOKING TIP: To save time, you can cook big batches of ground beef in advance, and store in 1-pound servings in the freezer.

Per Serving: Calories: 596; Total Fat: 17g; Saturated Fat: 6g; Cholesterol: 82mg; Sodium: 542mg; Carbohydrates: 79g; Fiber: 4g; Protein: 35g

Zucchini Lasagna

MAKE AHEAD

SERVES 8 / PREP TIME: 15 MINUTES / COOK TIME: 1 HOUR

Lasagna is a warm and comforting meal, but traditional lasagnas are very high in FODMAPs. We made our lasagna low-FODMAP by using low-FODMAP noodles and a tomato sauce without garlic or onion and by limiting the amount of cottage cheese or ricotta. We also replaced some of the noodles with zucchini to increase the nutrition. Laying the zucchini slices on towels is essential because it will help remove excess liquid, so the lasagna doesn't get watery. Extra lasagna slices will stay good in the freezer for up to 3 months.

Nonstick cooking spray, for greasing

1 small zucchini, peeled and sliced

1 pound lean ground beef

1 red bell pepper, chopped

2¾ cups tomato sauce

6 cooked low-FODMAP lasagna noodles

1 cup cottage cheese or ricotta cheese, divided

1½ cups shredded mozzarella cheese

¼ cup grated Parmesan cheese

1. Preheat the oven to 350°F. Grease a 9-by-13-inch baking dish.

2. Trim the ends of the zucchini, and, using a peeler, shave into thin slices. Lay the slices on a kitchen towel or paper towel, and let sit for at least 5 minutes. Use another towel to wipe off any liquid that seeps out the top.

3. Heat a large skillet over medium-high heat, and spray with cooking spray.

4. Add the beef and bell pepper, and cook for 8 to 10 minutes, or until the beef has browned. Carefully drain off and discard any fat.

5. Stir in the tomato sauce, and simmer for 5 minutes, or until slightly thickened.

6. Spread one-third of the meat sauce into the bottom of the prepared baking dish.

7. Layer 3 lasagna noodles, ½ cup of cottage cheese, half of the zucchini slices, and one-third of the meat sauce. Repeat the layers one more time with the remaining ingredients. Cover with aluminum foil.

> CONTINUED ON NEXT PAGE

8. Transfer the baking dish to the oven, bake for 35 minutes, then carefully remove and discard the foil, and sprinkle on the mozzarella and Parmesan cheeses. Return to the oven, and bake for 10 minutes, or until the cheese is melted and lightly browned. Remove from the oven.

9. Store leftovers in the refrigerator for up to 5 days.

VARIATION TIP: Add extra fiber by stirring 1 cup cooked lentils into the beef sauce.

FODMAP TIP: The low-FODMAP serving is one-eighth of the recipe. Cottage cheese and ricotta cheese are both low-FODMAP at 2 tablespoons each. Lactose-free versions of cottage cheese and ricotta cheese are FODMAP-free. If you can find a lactose-free version, you can use extra cottage cheese or ricotta and won't need to worry about the FODMAP serving size.

Per Serving: Calories: 343; Total Fat: 12g; Saturated Fat: 6g; Cholesterol: 59mg; Sodium: 327mg; Carbohydrates: 31g; Fiber: 2g; Protein: 26g

Slow Cooker Beef Stew

GLUTEN-FREE • MAKE AHEAD

SERVES 4 / PREP TIME: 10 MINUTES / COOK TIME: 8 HOURS

We knew we had to include a slow cooker stew recipe in this book. It's so nice to throw everything into the slow cooker and come back to a finished meal. Lauren likes using her Instant Pot® because you can brown the beef in the pot on the Sauté setting and don't have to use a skillet. Browning is important to maximize the flavor.

1 pound beef for stew, cut into
   1-inch pieces

5 medium carrots, peeled and chopped

2 medium potatoes, peeled and chopped

1 cup tomato juice

1 cup Nourishing Vegetable Broth
   (page 178) or low-FODMAP beef broth

½ cup finely chopped fennel bulb

½ cup finely chopped scallions, green
   parts only

1 teaspoon ground basil

Salt

Freshly ground black pepper

1 tablespoon cornstarch

1 tablespoon cold water

1. In a large nonstick skillet, over medium-high heat, sear the beef for 3 to 5 minutes, or until browned.

2. In a slow cooker, combine the beef, carrots, potatoes, tomato juice, broth, fennel, scallions, and basil. Season with salt and pepper. Cover, and cook on low for 8 hours.

3. In a small bowl, mix the cornstarch with the water, and stir well. Stir into the stew, let thicken for a few minutes, and serve.

VARIATION TIP: You can use 2 parsnips instead of 2 of the carrots.

COOKING TIP: Add another tablespoon of cornstarch if you want the gravy to be thicker.

Per Serving: Calories: 294; Total Fat: 7g; Saturated Fat: 2g; Cholesterol: 75mg; Sodium: 73mg; Carbohydrates: 31g; Fiber: 5g; Protein: 28g

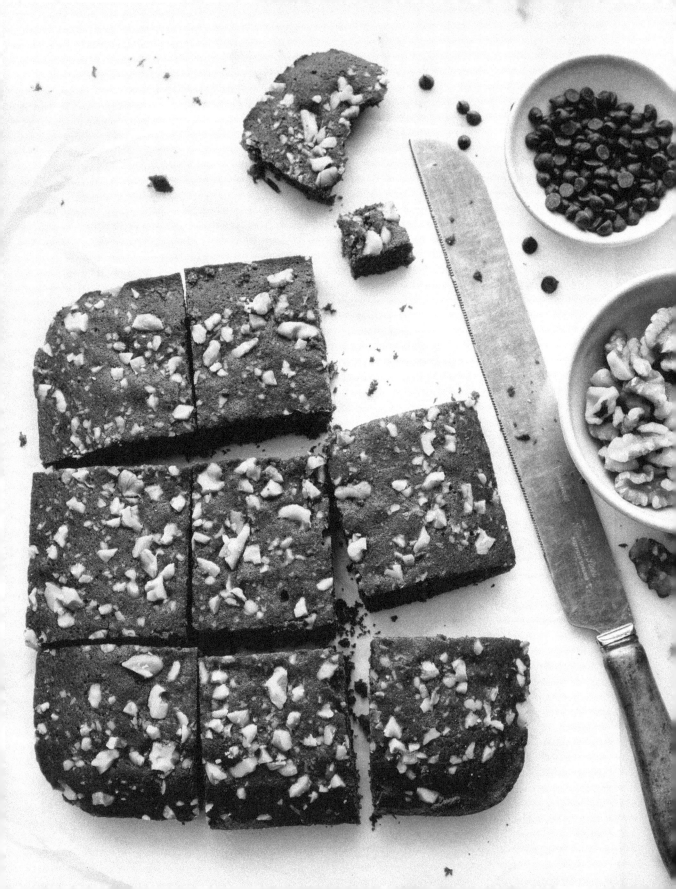

CHAPTER NINE

Snacks and Desserts

Chocolate-Walnut Brownies, page 169

Trail Mix

VEGETARIAN · 30 MINUTES OR LESS · MAKE AHEAD · ONE POT

SERVES 4 / PREP TIME: 5 MINUTES

Trail mix can help you survive in the wilderness . . . and survive your first few weeks on the low-FODMAP diet. A handful of trail mix can be a lifesaver when your stomach is rumbling and you need something in a hurry. The protein content and portability make it a great snack. Trail mix is an easy alternative to granola bars. Keep a batch in your pantry or in your desk at work.

¾ cup salted peanuts

½ cup Crispix cereal

½ cup chocolate chips

½ cup banana chips

¼ cup dried cranberries or raisins

In an airtight container, combine the peanuts, Crispix, chocolate chips, banana chips, and cranberries. Store in a cool, dry area for up to 2 weeks.

VARIATION TIP: Instead of peanuts, you can use pecans, walnuts, or macadamia nuts.

COOKING TIP: Double the batch so you have it handy throughout the week.

FODMAP TIP: A low-FODMAP serving is a quarter of the recipe. Once it is mixed, portion the trail mix into 4 ready-to-go plastic bags or containers.

Per Serving: Calories: 325; Total Fat: 20g; Saturated Fat: 6g; Cholesterol: 0mg; Sodium: 111mg; Carbohydrates: 33g; Fiber: 3g; Protein: 9g

No-Bake Bars

VEGETARIAN · 30 MINUTES OR LESS · MAKE AHEAD

MAKES 16 BARS [1 SERVING = 2 SQUARES] / PREP TIME: 10 MINUTES, PLUS 15 MINUTES IN THE FREEZER

There is a secret ingredient in these bars: raw quinoa. That's right: You can eat quinoa without cooking it. Raw quinoa has a surprisingly lovely crunch, and trust us, you won't break your teeth. We are keen on loading up snacks with as much nutrition as possible. Quinoa adds a great source of protein and fiber to these bars.

½ **cup brown rice syrup**

½ **cup natural peanut butter**

1 **tablespoon butter**

¼ **teaspoon salt**

1 **teaspoon vanilla extract**

4 **cups puffed rice cereal**

¼ **cup quinoa**

1. Line an 8-inch square baking dish with parchment paper.
2. In a large pot, combine the rice syrup, peanut butter, butter, and salt. Cook over medium heat until melted and easy to stir. Remove from the heat.
3. Stir in the vanilla, then add the cereal and quinoa. Stir gently to make sure that all of the cereal is mixed in.
4. Transfer the mixture to the prepared baking dish, and spread out evenly. Cover with another larger piece of parchment paper, and press very firmly with your hands or a pastry roller.
5. Place the baking dish in the freezer for 15 minutes. This allows the mixture to stick together so the bars can be cut without falling apart.
6. Pop the mixture out of the baking dish, and cut into 16 squares. Store in an airtight container in the refrigerator for 5 to 7 days.

SUBSTITUTION TIP: For a nut-free version, try sunflower seed butter instead of peanut butter.

COOKING TIP: Make a double batch, and store the squares in the freezer.

VARIATION TIP: Drizzle melted chocolate on top for a nice treat.

FODMAP TIP: A low-FODMAP serving is 2 squares.

Per Serving (2 squares): Calories: 216; Total Fat: 10g; Saturated Fat: 3g; Cholesterol: 4mg; Sodium: 103mg; Carbohydrates: 28g; Fiber: 2g; Protein: 7g

Flourless Peanut Butter–Banana Cookies

**VEGETARIAN · GLUTEN-FREE · 5 INGREDIENTS OR LESS ·
30 MINUTES OR LESS · MAKE AHEAD · ONE POT**

MAKES 27 COOKIES [3 COOKIES = 1 SERVING] / PREP TIME: 10 MINUTES / COOK TIME: 15 MINUTES

Audrey believes that cookies can be an "everyday" food. Therefore, these are a healthier version of classic peanut butter cookies. These cookies are naturally sweetened with a banana and are a good source of protein. Once the cookies cool, be ready with a cup of ice cold lactose-free milk or almond milk, and enjoy.

1 medium unripe banana

1 cup natural peanut butter

1 large egg

⅓ cup lightly packed brown sugar

1 teaspoon baking soda

¼ cup milk chocolate chips (optional)

1. Preheat the oven to 350°F. Line a sheet pan with parchment paper.

2. Place the banana on a plate or flat surface, and mash with a fork until it is puréed.

3. In a medium bowl, combine the mashed banana, peanut butter, egg, sugar, and baking soda. Mix with a fork until well combined. Add the chocolate chips (if using).

4. Leaving about 2 inches of space between each cookie, drop tablespoons of cookie dough onto the prepared sheet pan. You should have 27 small cookies.

5. Transfer the sheet pan to the oven. Bake for 12 minutes, or until the cookies are cooked in the middle. Remove from the oven, and let cool on a wire rack.

COOKING TIP: Make a double batch, and store leftovers in the freezer.

Per Serving (3 cookies): Calories: 218; Total Fat: 15g; Saturated Fat: 2g; Cholesterol: 21mg; Sodium: 154mg; Carbohydrates: 14g; Fiber: 2g; Protein: 10g

Roasted Red Pepper Hummus

VEGAN · GLUTEN-FREE · 30 MINUTES OR LESS · MAKE AHEAD · ONE POT

SERVES 6 [1 SERVING = ¼ CUP] / PREP TIME: 10 MINUTES

Audrey was once told by a Lebanese friend that the secret to making hummus the traditional way is to cream the tahini with lemon juice first. Once combined, you can add the rest of the ingredients. The red peppers make this hummus taste rich and a bit sweet. As with all chickpea recipes, you need to keep your eye on the serving size (see the FODMAP Tip).

**2 tablespoons freshly squeezed
lemon juice**

1 tablespoon tahini

1½ cups chickpeas, drained and rinsed

¾ cup jarred roasted red peppers, drained

**¼ cup chopped scallions, green
parts only**

**¼ cup coarsely chopped fresh basil or
1 tablespoon dried basil**

**1 tablespoon Garlic-Infused Oil
(page 184) or extra-virgin olive oil**

Pinch salt

Freshly ground black pepper

1. In a small bowl, using a fork, mix the lemon juice and tahini vigorously, until the tahini becomes creamy.

2. In a food processor, combine the lemon juice–tahini mixture, chickpeas, peppers, scallions, basil, and oil. Season with the salt and pepper. Blend until smooth.

COOKING TIP: Keeps in the refrigerator for 1 week.

FODMAP TIP: A low-FODMAP serving is ¼ cup.

Per Serving (¼ cup): Calories: 111; Total Fat: 5g; Saturated Fat: 1g; Cholesterol: 0mg; Sodium: 89mg; Carbohydrates: 14g; Fiber: 4g; Protein: 4g

Olive Lover's Hummus

VEGAN · GLUTEN-FREE · 5 INGREDIENTS OR LESS ·
30 MINUTES OR LESS · MAKE AHEAD · ONE POT

SERVES 6 / PREP TIME: 5 MINUTES

I think that we were pretty clever to come up with a hummus recipe that is low-FODMAP enough to enjoy a decent serving (see the FODMAP Tip below). Many people think that making low-FODMAP hummus is nearly impossible, so we set out to prove them wrong. This recipe is super-fast and pleasingly versatile. Enjoy it with cucumber, carrots, red bell peppers, or low-FODMAP crackers.

1½ cups canned chickpeas, drained
    and rinsed

½ cup pitted Kalamata olives

¼ cup coarsely chopped fresh basil
    leaves or 1 tablespoon dried
    basil leaves

2 tablespoons Garlic-Infused Oil
    (page 184) or extra-virgin olive oil, plus
    more as needed

In a food processor, combine the chickpeas, olives, basil, and oil. Pulse until it is well mixed. Drizzle with additional oil, if desired.

COOKING TIP: Snip the basil with a clean pair of scissors rather than chopping with a knife and cutting board so there is less to wash.

INGREDIENT TIP: Try using green pitted olives instead of Kalamata.

VARIATION TIP: Blend it to be smooth like hummus, or leave it chunky like tapenade.

FODMAP TIP: A low-FODMAP serving is ¼ cup.

Per Serving: Calories: 120; Total Fat: 7g; Saturated Fat: 1g; Cholesterol: 0mg; Sodium: 101mg; Carbohydrates: 12g; Fiber: 4g; Protein: 4g

Berry Yogurt Popsicles

VEGETARIAN · GLUTEN-FREE · 5 INGREDIENTS OR LESS · MAKE AHEAD · ONE POT

SERVES 2 / PREP TIME: 5 MINUTES / CHILL TIME: 2 HOURS

We had to include a healthy ice pop recipe to help you cool off in warm weather. You don't need to use a blender, so cleanup is easy. Use a plastic ice pop mold if you have one. If not, you can use an ice cube tray and toothpicks, or ice pop sticks cut in half.

½ cup chopped strawberries

¼ cup raspberries

1 tablespoon maple syrup

¾ cup lactose-free plain yogurt

1. In a bowl, use a fork to mash the strawberries and raspberries with the maple syrup. Stir in the yogurt.
2. Fill the ice pop molds. Freeze for at least 2 hours, or until solid.

COOKING TIP: If you use an ice cube tray instead of an ice pop mold, scoop in the yogurt mixture and then cover it with foil or plastic wrap. Poke toothpicks or ice pop sticks into the center of the foil or wrap and then freeze.

VARIATION TIP: You can use flavored lactose-free yogurt instead of the maple syrup and plain yogurt, or try sliced blueberries instead of the raspberries.

Per Serving: Calories: 110; Total Fat: 1g; Saturated Fat: 1g; Cholesterol: 6mg; Sodium: 66mg; Carbohydrates: 18g; Fiber: 2g; Protein: 6g

Chocolate Rounds with Nuts and Dried Fruit

VEGAN • GLUTEN-FREE • 5 INGREDIENTS OR LESS • 30 MINUTES OR LESS • MAKE AHEAD • ONE POT

MAKES 12 ROUNDS [1 SERVING = 3 ROUNDS] / PREP TIME: 5 MINUTES, PLUS 5 MINUTES TO COOL

These chocolate rounds look fancy, but they are so easy to make! Just melt the chocolate and sprinkle your toppings of choice on top. We like the combination of walnuts and raisins, but you can use any low-FODMAP nuts and dried fruit you prefer. You can make them look festive in December using dried cranberries and pumpkin seeds.

½ cup (4 ounces) chopped dark chocolate

¼ cup chopped walnuts

¼ cup Thompson raisins

Pinch sea salt (optional)

1. Line a large plate with parchment paper.
2. In a microwave-safe bowl, microwave the chocolate for 30 seconds and then stir. Repeat in 30-second increments for 90 to 120 seconds total, or until the chocolate has fully melted.
3. Scoop the melted chocolate onto the parchment paper, making 12 circles each about ½ inch wide.
4. Sprinkle the walnuts, raisins, and salt (if using) on top, and gently press into the chocolate. Wait at least 5 minutes for the chocolate to harden and then enjoy.

COOKING TIP: If you make extra chocolate rounds, you can store them in the refrigerator or freezer so that they are ready whenever you need a sweet treat.

VARIATION TIP: Switch it up and try peanuts, pecans, almonds, hazelnuts, macadamia nuts, pumpkin seeds, sunflower seeds, dried cranberries, or shredded coconut. A sprinkle of cinnamon instead of sea salt is also tasty. You can also try with white or milk chocolate instead of dark chocolate (see FODMAP Tip below).

FODMAP TIP: When made with dark chocolate, a low-FODMAP serving is 3 rounds. If made with white or milk chocolate, a low-FODMAP serving is 2 rounds.

Per Serving (3 rounds): Calories: 224; Total Fat: 15g; Saturated Fat: 7g; Cholesterol: 0mg; Sodium: 1mg; Carbohydrates: 21g; Fiber: 3g; Protein: 2g

Tzatziki Dip

VEGETARIAN · GLUTEN-FREE · 30 MINUTES OR LESS · MAKE AHEAD · ONE POT

MAKES ½ CUP [1 SERVING = 2 TABLESPOONS] / PREP TIME: 5 MINUTES

This tzatziki dip makes eating vegetables fun. If you want to add garlic flavor, use freshly made Garlic-Infused Oil (page 184). If you don't like garlic, there is still lots of flavor from the cucumber, lemon, and dill.

2 tablespoons grated and drained cucumber

½ cup lactose-free plain Greek yogurt

1 teaspoon Garlic-Infused Oil (page 184) or extra-virgin olive oil, plus more as needed

1 teaspoon freshly squeezed lemon juice, plus more as needed

1 teaspoon dried dill or 1 tablespoon fresh dill, plus more as needed

⅛ teaspoon salt, plus more as needed

1/16 teaspoon freshly ground black pepper, plus more as needed

In a bowl, combine the cucumber, yogurt, oil, lemon juice, dill, salt, and pepper. Taste and add more oil, lemon juice, dill, salt, or pepper as desired. Enjoy right away, or store in an airtight container in the refrigerator for up to 3 days.

COOKING TIP: You can drain the grated cucumber by gently pressing it with a tea towel to help release the extra water. This step is important to make sure your dip isn't watery.

Per Serving (2 tablespoons):
Calories: 31; Total Fat: 2g; Saturated Fat: 0g; Cholesterol: 3mg; Sodium: 87mg; Carbohydrates: 1g; Fiber: 0g; Protein: 3g

Peanut Butter Power Balls

VEGAN · 30 MINUTES OR LESS · MAKE AHEAD · ONE POT

MAKES 24 BALLS [1 SERVING = 4 BALLS] / PREP TIME: 5 MINUTES, PLUS 10 MINUTES TO CHILL

These energy balls are an ideal on-the-go snack, can provide a quick energy boost, and are more nutritious than the average granola bar. Lauren originally made this recipe so she would have a filling snack to eat between classes. Audrey now loves making these for her kids.

⅓ cup peanut butter

6 tablespoons maple syrup

¾ teaspoon ground cinnamon

Pinch salt

⅓ cup rolled oats

6 tablespoons puffed rice

3 tablespoons chocolate chips

1. In a bowl, stir together the peanut butter, maple syrup, cinnamon, and salt until well combined. If your peanut butter is not mixing well, microwave it for 15 seconds or until soft and easy to stir.

2. Mix in the oats, puffed rice, and chocolate chips.

3. Grab a handful of the dough, and squeeze it together. Roll it into a ball shape about 1 inch in diameter, and place in a container. Repeat with the rest of the dough, making 24 small balls. Chill in the refrigerator or freezer for at least 10 minutes, or until they have hardened. Store in an airtight container for up to 1 week in the refrigerator or 3 months in the freezer.

COOKING TIP: Wet your hands with a bit of cold water to help avoid the dough sticking too much to your hands.

VARIATION TIP: The puffed rice can be puffed brown rice or Rice Krispies. You can also try shredded unsweetened coconut instead.

INGREDIENT TIP: Skip the salt if your peanut butter has added salt. Mini chocolate chips work even better than regular chocolate chips.

Per Serving (4 balls): Calories: 286; Total Fat: 14g; Saturated Fat: 4g; Cholesterol: 1mg; Sodium: 106mg; Carbohydrates: 35g; Fiber: 4g; Protein: 9g

Chocolate-Walnut Brownies

VEGETARIAN • 30 MINUTES OR LESS • ONE BOWL

MAKES 9 BROWNIES [1 BROWNIE = 1 SERVING] / PREP TIME: 10 MINUTES / COOK TIME: 20 MINUTES

Low-FODMAP and gluten-free baking seems to have a reputation for being difficult. Brownies are one of the easiest baked goods to make. Make sure to use an 8-inch square baking dish. Our main tip is don't overmix the batter. After adding the flour, stir just until all the flour is mixed in and then pour it into the pan. Overmixing can affect the texture.

Nonstick cooking spray, for greasing

8 tablespoons (1 stick) butter, melted

½ cup white sugar

¼ cup maple syrup

2 large eggs

1 teaspoon vanilla extract

½ cup cocoa powder

¾ teaspoon baking powder

¼ teaspoon sea salt

¾ cup low-FODMAP flour blend

¼ cup almond flour

¼ cup walnuts

¼ cup chocolate chips (optional)

1. Preheat the oven to 350°F. Grease an 8-inch square baking dish.
2. In a large bowl, mix together the butter, sugar, maple syrup, eggs, and vanilla.
3. Stir in the cocoa powder, baking powder, and salt.
4. Add the flour blend and almond flour, and stir until just combined.
5. Pour the batter into the prepared baking dish, and spread evenly.
6. Sprinkle walnuts and chocolate chips (if using) on top.
7. Transfer the baking dish to the oven, and bake for 20 minutes, or until the middle is cooked and no longer sticky. Remove from the oven, and let cool for at least 15 minutes before removing from the pan. Store in a container for a few days or freeze for up to 1 month.

COOKING TIP: Don't overbake the brownies, or they can become dry. Test the middle by sticking a butter knife in. If the knife comes out with wet batter stuck to it, bake it for a couple more minutes and then test again.

VARIATION TIP: Pecans are a nice alternative to walnuts.

Per Serving (1 brownie): Calories: 227; Total Fat: 13g; Saturated Fat: 7g; Cholesterol: 68mg; Sodium: 142mg; Carbohydrates: 28g; Fiber: 3g; Protein: 4g

Classic Chocolate Chip Cookies

VEGETARIAN • 30 MINUTES OR LESS • ONE POT

MAKES 36 COOKIES [1 SERVING = 4 COOKIES] / PREP TIME: 20 MINUTES / COOK TIME: 10 MINUTES

Becoming dietitians didn't erase our love for cookies. Having IBS doesn't mean you can't enjoy a treat occasionally.

8 tablespoons (1 stick) butter, softened

½ cup white sugar

½ cup packed brown sugar

1 large egg

1 teaspoon vanilla extract

¼ teaspoon salt

¾ cup plus 2 tablespoons low-FODMAP flour blend

¼ cup almond flour

½ teaspoon xanthan gum

½ teaspoon baking soda

¾ cup chocolate chips

1. Preheat the oven to 325°F. Line a sheet pan with parchment paper.
2. In a large bowl, using a fork, cream the butter, white sugar, and brown sugar until well combined.
3. Beat in the egg, vanilla, and salt.
4. In another bowl, whisk together the flour blend, almond flour, xanthan gum, and baking soda.
5. Slowly mix the flour mixture into the butter mixture until just combined.
6. Stir in the chocolate chips.
7. Chill the dough in the refrigerator or freezer for at least 10 minutes.
8. Leaving about 2 inches of space between each cookie, drop spoonfuls of the dough onto the prepared sheet pan. You should have 36 small cookies.
9. Transfer the sheet pan to the oven, and bake for 10 minutes, or until just lightly browned on the bottom and soft but firm on top. Remove from the oven. Let cool for at least 5 minutes on the sheet pan and then transfer to a cooling rack.

INGREDIENT TIP: You can use a commercially prepared low-FODMAP flour blend that is meant to be substituted 1-to-1 for all-purpose flour. Lauren prefers to make her own: ½ cup white rice flour, 3 tablespoons sweet or glutinous rice flour, and 3 tablespoons tapioca starch.

Per Serving (4 cookies): Calories: 397; Total Fat: 16g; Saturated Fat: 10g; Cholesterol: 51mg; Sodium: 257mg; Carbohydrates: 37g; Fiber: 2g; Protein: 3g

Banana-Carrot Muffins

VEGETARIAN • ONE POT

MAKES 12 MUFFINS [1 SERVING = 2 MUFFINS] / PREP TIME: 5 MINUTES / COOK TIME: 35 MINUTES

Lauren's two favorite types of muffins are banana and carrot, so these muffins truly are the best of both worlds. They are nicely browned on the outside but still soft and moist on the inside. Skipping muffin liners helps them to brown up nicely. As long as you grease the tin, the muffins will pop right out and make cleanup easy.

Nonstick cooking spray, for greasing

1½ cups packed grated carrots

1 cup mashed ripe bananas (2 medium bananas)

⅔ cup brown sugar

8 tablespoons (1 stick) butter, melted

½ cup lactose-free milk or almond milk

2 large eggs

1 teaspoon vanilla extract

1 cup plus 2 tablespoons low-FODMAP flour blend

⅔ cup rolled oats

½ cup almond meal

1 teaspoon baking soda

1 teaspoon ground cinnamon

½ teaspoon salt

1. Preheat the oven to 375°F. Grease a 12-cup muffin tin.

2. In a large bowl, mix together the carrots, bananas, sugar, butter, milk, eggs, and vanilla.

3. In a separate bowl, mix together the flour blend, oats, almond meal, baking soda, cinnamon, and salt.

4. Slowly mix the dry ingredients into the wet ingredients, and stir until just combined. Pour into the muffin tin.

5. Transfer the muffin tin to the oven, and bake for about 35 minutes, or until the tops are browned and firm. Remove from the oven.

6. Let the muffins cool in the pan for at least 5 minutes and then remove. They will stay fresh in a container at room temperature for a few days or in the freezer for a few months.

COOKING TIP: You can use paper liners, but the muffins may stick to them.

VARIATION TIP: For extra flavor, add ¼ teaspoon ground ginger, ¼ teaspoon nutmeg, or both to the batter. You can also mix in ¼ cup chopped walnuts, ¼ cup dried cranberries, or both.

Per Serving (2 muffins): Calories: 429; Total Fat: 22g; Saturated Fat: 11g; Cholesterol: 103mg; Sodium: 383mg; Carbohydrates: 52g; Fiber: 4g; Protein: 8g

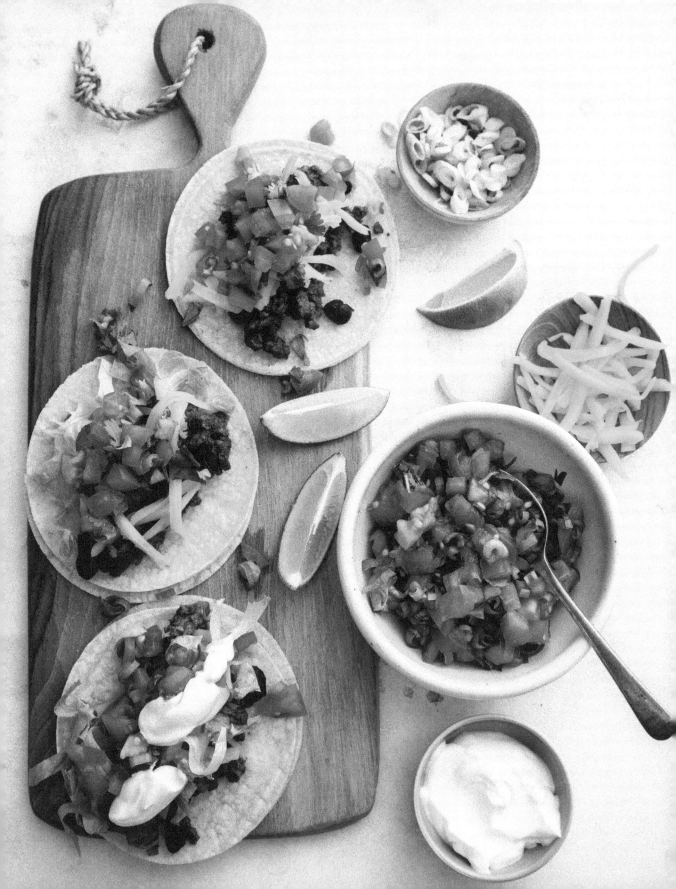

CHAPTER TEN

Broths, Sauces, Oils, and Dressings

Chile-Lime DIY Tacos (page 153) with Fresh Cut Salsa (page 177)

Sweet Barbecue Sauce

VEGAN · GLUTEN-FREE · 30 MINUTES OR LESS · MAKE AHEAD · ONE POT

MAKES ½ CUP [1 SERVING = 1 TABLESPOON] / PREP TIME: 5 MINUTES

This sauce is tangy and sweet, but what Audrey loves most is how quickly it comes together. Conventional barbecue sauce is riddled with high-FODMAP ingredients, but you can enjoy this one without worry. It goes well on pork, chicken, hamburgers, veggie burgers, and burritos.

½ cup light brown sugar

¼ cup tomato paste

3 tablespoons apple cider vinegar

1 teaspoon dry mustard

1 teaspoon smoked paprika

1 teaspoon freshly ground black pepper

¾ teaspoon salt

In a medium bowl, mix together the sugar, tomato paste, vinegar, mustard, paprika, pepper, and salt. Let sit for 10 minutes to allow the sugar to dissolve.

VARIATION TIP: You can try regular paprika with liquid smoke instead of smoked paprika. For a thinner sauce, add another 1 tablespoon vinegar. You can also use white vinegar instead of apple cider vinegar.

COOKING TIP: Double this recipe, and store the sauce in the refrigerator for 2 weeks.

Per Serving (1 tablespoon): Calories: 46; Total Fat: 0g; Saturated Fat: 0g; Cholesterol: 0mg; Sodium: 228mg; Carbohydrates: 11g; Fiber: 1g; Protein: 1g

Fresh Cut Salsa

VEGAN • GLUTEN-FREE • 5 INGREDIENTS OR LESS • 30 MINUTES OR LESS • MAKE AHEAD • ONE POT

SERVES 4 / PREP TIME: 10 MINUTES

You don't have to miss out on salsa while on the low-FODMAP diet. Salsa is traditionally made with fresh tomatoes, onion, cilantro, and lime. In our recipe, we simply substitute scallion greens for an onion bulb. Two of our recipes use this salsa: the Loaded Nachos (page 118) and the Chile-Lime DIY Tacos (page 153). You can also enjoy it with a simple bowl of tortilla chips.

4 tomatoes, chopped

5 scallions, green parts only, chopped

½ cup chopped fresh cilantro

Grated zest and juice of 1 lime

Pinch salt (optional)

In a medium bowl, combine the tomatoes, scallions, cilantro, and lime zest and juice. Season with salt (if using).

SUBSTITUTION TIP: Use fresh basil or parsley instead of cilantro. If you like it spicy, add ½ jalapeño pepper. Note that chile peppers are low-FODMAP but can be a digestive trigger for some people.

COOKING TIP: Prepare this salsa in advance, and store in the refrigerator for up to 5 days.

Per Serving: Calories: 34; Total Fat: 0g; Saturated Fat: 0g; Cholesterol: 0mg; Sodium: 10mg; Carbohydrates: 8g; Fiber: 3g; Protein: 2g

Nourishing Vegetable Broth

VEGAN • **GLUTEN-FREE** • **MAKE AHEAD** • **ONE POT**

MAKES 8 CUPS [1 SERVING = 1 CUP] / PREP TIME: 10 MINUTES / COOK TIME: 1 HOUR

This broth is like a multivitamin in your bowl. It is loaded with wholesome nutritious vegetables. We created this broth because it is difficult to find commercially made vegetarian broths that don't contain onions and garlic. We love that this broth adds so much nutrition to your meals.

1 cup coarsely chopped leeks or
    scallions, green parts only

3 carrots, roughly chopped

1 cup chopped oyster mushrooms

2 large kale leaves, coarsely chopped

8½ cups water, divided

2 large bay leaves

4 sprigs parsley

1 teaspoon salt

1. In a large pot, combine the leeks, carrots, mushrooms, and kale with ½ cup of water. Cook, covered, over medium-high heat for about 5 minutes, or until fork-tender.

2. Add the remaining water, bay leaves, parsley, and salt. Bring to a boil, then reduce the heat to a simmer and cook for 1 hour or longer. The longer it simmers, the better the flavor.

3. Line a sieve with 2 layers of cheesecloth, and place over a bowl. Strain the broth through the cheesecloth, squeezing the cloth in a bundle to remove all of the broth.

4. Store the broth as is, or reduce to 1 cup on the stove for a condensed version.

VARIATION TIP: Use any vegetables or peelings from any vegetables on the low-FODMAP list (see page 12).

COOKING TIP: If your refrigerator space comes at a premium, you can condense the broth to 1 cup and add water when it is time to use. You can also make a double recipe and store the extra in the freezer.

Per Serving (1 cup): Calories: 15; Total Fat: 0g; Saturated Fat: 0g; Cholesterol: 0mg; Sodium: 390mg; Carbohydrates: 4g; Fiber: 0g; Protein: 0g

Goddess Dressing

VEGAN • 5 INGREDIENTS OR LESS • 30 MINUTES OR LESS • MAKE AHEAD • ONE POT

MAKES 1 CUP [1 SERVING = 2 TABLESPOONS] / PREP TIME: 5 MINUTES

This is an Asian-style dressing made with nutritional yeast. It is popular among vegans because it has a rich umami flavor similar to Parmesan cheese, and it is a great source of B-complex vitamins. We recommend using this dressing on the Forbidden Edamame Bowl (page 125) and the Tofu Noodle Bowl (page 114). It's also a great salad dressing on mixed greens or wilted spinach. Audrey likes it so much she could practically drink it with a straw.

¼ **cup rice-wine vinegar**

¼ **cup nutritional yeast**

¼ **cup water**

¼ **cup soy sauce**

2 tablespoons extra-virgin olive oil or
   sesame oil

In a salad dressing shaker, combine the vinegar, nutritional yeast, water, soy sauce, and oil. Shake well to emulsify.

COOKING TIP: Store the dressing in the refrigerator for up to 2 weeks.

VARIATION TIP: You can use apple cider vinegar instead of rice-wine vinegar.

Per Serving (2 tablespoons):
Calories: 69; Total Fat: 4g; Saturated Fat: 1g; Cholesterol: 0mg; Sodium: 452mg; Carbohydrates: 4g; Fiber: 2g; Protein: 5g

The Perfect Pesto

VEGETARIAN · GLUTEN-FREE · 30 MINUTES OR LESS · MAKE AHEAD · ONE POT

MAKES 1 CUP [1 SERVING = 2 TABLESPOONS] / PREP TIME: 10 MINUTES

This pesto is suitably named "perfect," as it is delicious and reliably low-FODMAP, and you won't have to worry about embarrassing garlic breath after eating it. We are sure you will enjoy it on a warm plate of low-FODMAP pasta. This pesto is also a great accompaniment to the Prosciutto-Wrapped Chicken (page 145).

2 cups packed basil leaves

⅓ cup pine nuts or walnuts

½ cup grated Parmesan cheese

1 tablespoon freshly squeezed lemon juice

Pinch salt

½ cup Garlic-Infused Oil (page 184) or extra-virgin olive oil

1. In a food processor, combine the basil and pine nuts, and pulse until well blended.

2. Add the cheese, lemon juice, and salt.

3. While the machine is running, slowly pour in the oil. Blend until smooth.

COOKING TIP: Pesto can be stored in the refrigerator for 3 days. You can also freeze it in a freezer bag and simply break off chunks when you are ready to use it. Pesto will keep for up to a month in the freezer.

Per Serving (2 tablespoons):
Calories: 182; Total Fat: 19g; Saturated Fat: 3g; Cholesterol: 5mg; Sodium: 8mg; Carbohydrates: 1g; Fiber: 0g; Protein: 3g

Maple–Balsamic Vinegar Dressing

VEGAN • GLUTEN-FREE • 5 INGREDIENTS OR LESS •
30 MINUTES OR LESS • MAKE AHEAD • ONE POT

MAKES ½ CUP [1 SERVING = 1 TABLESPOON] / PREP TIME: 5 MINUTES

This is a handy everyday dressing to have in your refrigerator for mixed greens, spinach salad, or coleslaw. We use it for the Warm Roasted Vegetable Salad (page 104) and the Kale Salad (page 94). We are sure that you will find many other uses for it, too.

¼ cup Garlic-Infused Oil (page 184) or
   extra-virgin olive oil

2 tablespoons balsamic vinegar

1 tablespoon maple syrup

1 teaspoon Dijon mustard

½ teaspoon salt (optional)

½ teaspoon freshly ground black pepper

In a salad dressing shaker, combine the oil, vinegar, maple syrup, mustard, salt (if using), and pepper. Shake well to emulsify.

VARIATION TIP: Try lemon juice, apple cider vinegar, or rice vinegar instead of balsamic vinegar.

COOKING TIP: Purchase a salad dressing shaker or two to store your homemade salad dressings. If you don't have one, a Mason jar or other storage container with a lid will work just as well.

COOKING TIP: Double this recipe, and store it in the refrigerator for up to 2 weeks.

Per Serving (1 tablespoon):
Calories: 62; Total Fat: 6g; Saturated Fat: 1g; Cholesterol: 0mg; Sodium: 8mg; Carbohydrates: 2g; Fiber: 0g; Protein: 0g

Creamy Dipping Duo

**VEGETARIAN · GLUTEN-FREE · 5 INGREDIENTS OR LESS ·
30 MINUTES OR LESS · MAKE AHEAD · ONE POT**

MAKES 1 TABLESPOON [1 SERVING = 1 TABLESPOON] / PREP TIME: 5 MINUTES

We couldn't decide which of our favorite sauces to include in this book, so we are giving both of them to you! There's no reason why the low-FODMAP diet should be bland and flavorless when you can enjoy these amazing dips. You can choose between spicy and mild.

FOR THE SPICY SRIRACHA MAYONNAISE

1 tablespoon mayonnaise

1 teaspoon sriracha

FOR THE MILD CURRY MAYONNAISE

**1 tablespoon mayonnaise or lactose-free
   Greek yogurt**

**¼ teaspoon curry powder (no onion
   or garlic)**

In a small bowl, mix together the mayonnaise with the sriracha or the curry powder.

VARIATION TIP: Use lactose-free plain Greek yogurt instead of mayonnaise (or use half yogurt and half mayonnaise).

COOKING TIP: Make extra, and store it in an airtight container in the refrigerator for up to 4 days.

FODMAP TIP: Monash tested sriracha and found that it has a low-FODMAP serving size. One serving of the Spicy Sriracha Mayonnaise is low-FODMAP. However, chile peppers may be a digestive trigger for some people.

SPICY SRIRACHA MAYONNAISE
Per Serving (1 tablespoon):
Calories: 95; Total Fat: 10g; Saturated Fat: 2g; Cholesterol: 5mg; Sodium: 125mg; Carbohydrates: 1g; Fiber: 0g; Protein: 0g

MILD CURRY MAYONNAISE
Per Serving (1 tablespoon):
Calories: 92; Total Fat: 10g; Saturated Fat: 2g; Cholesterol: 5mg; Sodium: 90mg; Carbohydrates: 0g; Fiber: 0g; Protein: 0g

Strawberry-Lemon Chia Seed Jam

VEGAN · GLUTEN-FREE · 5 INGREDIENTS OR LESS ·
30 MINUTES OR LESS · MAKE AHEAD · ONE POT

MAKES 2 CUPS [1 SERVING = 2 TABLESPOONS] / PREP TIME: 5 MINUTES / COOK TIME: 25 MINUTES

We have loosely called this recipe a jam, but it's really so much more. Audrey's favorite way to enjoy it is in a bowl of lactose-free yogurt and Sunshine Granola (page 72). It is also delicious on buttered low-FODMAP toast or as a topping on oatmeal or pancakes. With all of these options, you should consider doubling the batch.

4 cups strawberries, fresh or frozen

¼ cup maple syrup

2 tablespoons chia seeds

1 tablespoon freshly squeezed
  lemon juice

1. In a medium pot, combine the strawberries, maple syrup, and chia seeds. Bring to a rolling boil over medium-high heat.

2. Reduce the heat to medium-low, and cook for 10 minutes, stirring occasionally so the mixture doesn't burn on the bottom of the pan, or until it has thickened a little. Remove from the heat.

3. Mash the berries with a potato masher or potato ricer if you like a smoother jam. Add the lemon juice.

4. Boil the jam for another 10 minutes, or until reduced to 2 cups.

5. Pour the jam into 2 (1-cup) jars. Let the jam cool completely before closing the jars with lids. The jam will thicken as it cools.

COOKING TIP: This jam will keep for 7 to 10 days in the refrigerator or more than 3 months in the freezer.

Per Serving (2 tablespoons):
Calories: 34; Total Fat: 1g; Saturated Fat: 0g; Cholesterol: 0mg; Sodium: 1mg; Carbohydrates: 7g; Fiber: 1g; Protein: 1g

Garlic-Infused Oil

VEGAN • GLUTEN-FREE • 5 INGREDIENTS OR LESS •
30 MINUTES OR LESS • MAKE AHEAD • ONE POT

MAKES ¼ CUP [1 SERVING = 1 TABLESPOON] / PREP TIME: 1 MINUTE / COOK TIME: 5 MINUTES

This Garlic-Infused Oil is full of amazing garlic flavor without the FODMAPs! When garlic is heated in oil, its flavors blend with the oil, but the FODMAPs remain in the garlic. By removing the garlic, the oil that is left behind is low-FODMAP. Please note that this rule does not apply when cooking garlic in water or water-containing foods (such as broth or vegetables) because the FODMAPs will dissolve into water and can't be removed by simply taking out the garlic pieces. Homemade garlic oil is not shelf stable, so it is essential that you keep this oil in the refrigerator to avoid the risk of botulism poisoning. Always label the containers of infused oils, and wash them well before and after using.

¼ cup extra-virgin olive oil

2 garlic cloves, quartered

1. In a small skillet, heat the oil over medium-low heat.
2. Once the oil is hot, add the garlic. Stir, and simmer for a few minutes, or until the oil is fragrant and the garlic has browned.
3. Using a spoon, remove all of the garlic. Store the oil in the refrigerator for up to 3 days.

FODMAP TIP: It is essential to remove all pieces of garlic, which can typically be removed with a spoon. If there are any small garlic pieces left, use a fine-mesh strainer or cheesecloth to strain the oil.

COOKING TIP: You can use the flat side of a large chef's knife to crush the garlic cloves, making them easier to peel.

INGREDIENT TIP: Olive oil will solidify when stored in the refrigerator. When it's brought back to room temperature, it will become liquid again.

VARIATION TIP: Other mild-tasting oils can be used, such as canola or sunflower.

Per Serving (1 tablespoon):
Calories: 120; Total Fat: 14g; Saturated Fat: 2g; Cholesterol: 0mg; Sodium: 0mg; Carbohydrates: 0g; Fiber: 0g; Protein: 0g

Onion-Infused Oil

VEGAN • GLUTEN-FREE • 5 INGREDIENTS OR LESS •
30 MINUTES OR LESS • MAKE AHEAD • ONE POT

MAKES ¼ CUP [1 SERVING = 1 TABLESPOON] / PREP TIME: 1 MINUTE / COOK TIME: 5 MINUTES

Just like our Garlic-Infused Oil, this Onion-Infused Oil is full of amazing flavor but doesn't contain any of the FODMAPs. This oil is not shelf stable, so it's essential that this oil is kept in the refrigerator to avoid the risk of botulism poisoning. It will keep for up to 3 days. Always label the containers of infused oils, and wash them well before and after using.

¼ small onion, cut into 8 pieces

¼ cup extra-virgin olive oil

1. In a small skillet, heat the oil over medium-low heat.
2. Once the oil is hot, add the onion. Stir, and simmer for a few minutes, or until the oil is fragrant and the onion has browned.
3. Remove all of the onion. Store the oil in the refrigerator for up to 3 days.

FODMAP TIP: It's essential to remove all pieces of onion. If there are any small onion pieces left, use a fine-mesh strainer or cheesecloth to strain the oil.

INGREDIENT TIP: Olive oil will solidify when stored in the refrigerator. When it's brought back to room temperature, it will become liquid again.

VARIATION TIP: Other mild-tasting oils can be used, such as canola or sunflower. You can also make oil infused with both garlic and onion.

Per Serving (1 tablespoon):
Calories: 120; Total Fat: 14g; Saturated Fat: 2g; Cholesterol: 0mg; Sodium: 0mg; Carbohydrates: 0g; Fiber: 0g; Protein: 0g

Cajun Spice Mix

VEGAN • GLUTEN-FREE • 30 MINUTES OR LESS • MAKE AHEAD • ONE POT

MAKES ¼ CUP [1 SERVING = 1 TEASPOON] / PREP TIME: 1 MINUTE

Many store-bought spice mixes contain garlic and onion. Luckily, it takes only a minute to make your own. The flavors of this Cajun blend combine nicely with our homemade Garlic-Infused Oil (page 184). We use this mix in our Cajun-Spiced Root Vegetable Fries (page 103) and Fish in a Bag (page 139). We also like keeping extra in our cupboard to add to other recipes as we please.

1 tablespoon smoked paprika or paprika

1 tablespoon dried oregano

1 tablespoon brown or white sugar

2 teaspoons dried thyme

½ teaspoon salt

½ teaspoon freshly ground black pepper

⅛ teaspoon cayenne

In a storage container, spice shaker, or Mason jar, combine the paprika, oregano, sugar, thyme, salt, pepper, and cayenne. Cover and store at room temperature.

VARIATION TIP: If you can tolerate spicy foods without triggering IBS symptoms, you can try increasing the amount of cayenne. If you want extra chile flavor without the spice, add 1 teaspoon ancho chile powder, which is very mild.

Per Serving (1 teaspoon): Calories: 7; Total Fat: 0g; Saturated Fat: 0g; Cholesterol: 0mg; Sodium: 97mg; Carbohydrates: 2g; Fiber: 1g; Protein: 0g

Cranberry Vinaigrette

VEGAN · GLUTEN-FREE · 30 MINUTES OR LESS · MAKE AHEAD · ONE POT

MAKES ½ CUP [1 SERVING = 2 TABLESPOONS] / PREP TIME: 1 MINUTE / COOK TIME: 15 MINUTES

We like using this sweet and simple vinaigrette in our Cranberry-Quinoa Salad (page 100) and on any mixed green salad. Simmering the cranberry juice helps to concentrate it so you get a burst of cranberry flavor.

½ cup 100 percent cranberry juice

1 tablespoon extra-virgin olive oil

1 tablespoon red-wine vinegar

1 tablespoon maple syrup

⅛ teaspoon salt

⅛ teaspoon freshly ground black pepper

1. In a small saucepan, bring the cranberry juice to a boil.
2. Reduce the heat to low, and simmer for 10 minutes, or until reduced by about one-third. Remove from the heat, and let cool.
3. Whisk in the oil, vinegar, maple syrup, salt, and pepper. Store in an airtight container in the refrigerator for up to 2 weeks.

FODMAP TIP: Cranberry juice is low-FODMAP; however, you will need to read the ingredient list very carefully and avoid the ones that contain added fruit juices (such as apple) or high-FODMAP sweeteners (such as high-fructose corn syrup or glucose-fructose).

Per Serving (2 tablespoons):
Calories: 38; Total Fat: 2g; Saturated Fat: 0g; Cholesterol: 0mg; Sodium: 38mg; Carbohydrates: 6g; Fiber: 0g; Protein: 0g

Caesar Vinaigrette

GLUTEN-FREE · 30 MINUTES OR LESS · MAKE AHEAD · ONE POT

MAKES ½ CUP [1 SERVING = 2 TABLESPOONS PER SERVING] / PREP TIME: 5 MINUTES

Our Caesar dressing has all of the flavor without any of the fructans. Many people who start the low-FODMAP diet think they have to give up garlic-y Caesar salad. Lauren was able to modify her mom's vinaigrette and use Garlic-Infused Oil (page 184) instead of garlic cloves to make a flavorful vinaigrette.

⅓ cup Garlic-Infused Oil (page 184)

1 tablespoon liquid pasteurized egg white or mayonnaise

1 tablespoon red-wine vinegar

1 tablespoon freshly squeezed lemon juice

1 teaspoon freshly ground black pepper

¼ teaspoon anchovy paste

¼ teaspoon smooth Dijon mustard or ⅛ teaspoon dry mustard powder

1 drop Tabasco sauce (optional)

1. In a food processor or high-powered blender, combine the Garlic-Infused Oil and egg white, and blend.

2. Add the vinegar, lemon juice, pepper, anchovy paste, mustard, and Tabasco (if using). Pulse to combine.

3. Store the extra dressing in an airtight container in the refrigerator for up to 3 days. Mix again before using.

SUBSTITUTION TIP: Omit the anchovy to make it vegetarian, and use vegan mayonnaise instead of egg white to make it vegan.

INGREDIENT TIP: Raw egg whites are traditionally used in Caesar salad but may contain salmonella. Our food-safe version uses liquid pasteurized egg whites or mayonnaise. Look for pasteurized egg whites, which are sold in paper cartons, in the dairy and egg section of your grocery store.

Per Serving (2 tablespoons):
Calories: 167; Total Fat: 19g; Saturated Fat: 2g; Cholesterol: 1mg; Sodium: 26mg; Carbohydrates: 1g; Fiber: 0g; Protein: 1g

Orange-Ginger Marinade

VEGAN • 30 MINUTES OR LESS • MAKE AHEAD • ONE POT

MAKES 1½ CUPS [1 SERVING = 2 TABLESPOONS] / PREP TIME: 5 MINUTES / COOK TIME: 10 MINUTES

Freshly squeezed orange juice and grated ginger are the highlights of this marinade. We use it in our Pork Tenderloin Medallions (page 150), but it also is great for chicken. Lauren adapted this recipe from her parents' favorite marinade recipe.

½ **cup soy sauce**

½ **cup freshly squeezed orange juice (about 2 oranges)**

¼ **cup Garlic-Infused Oil (page 184) or extra-virgin olive oil**

4 teaspoons grated peeled fresh ginger or 2 teaspoons ground ginger

1 tablespoon brown sugar

2 teaspoons smooth Dijon mustard or 1 teaspoon dry mustard

1 teaspoon salt

¼ **teaspoon freshly ground black pepper**

In a medium saucepan, combine the soy sauce, orange juice, oil, ginger, sugar, mustard, salt, and pepper. Bring to a boil over high heat, then reduce the heat to low and simmer for 5 minutes, or until thickened slightly. Remove from the heat, and let cool. Store any leftover sauce in an airtight container in the refrigerator for up to 3 days.

COOKING TIP: Make fresh Garlic-Infused Oil (page 184) in the saucepan, and remove all garlic pieces. Then, add the other marinade ingredients and cook, so you have only one pan to clean up.

Per Serving (2 tablespoons):
Calories: 55; Total Fat: 5g; Saturated Fat: 1g; Cholesterol: 0mg; Sodium: 797mg; Carbohydrates: 3g; Fiber: 0g; Protein: 1g

Poppy Seed Salad Dressing

VEGAN · GLUTEN-FREE · 30 MINUTES OR LESS · MAKE AHEAD · ONE POT

MAKES ¼ CUP [1 SERVING = 1 TABLESPOON] / PREP TIME: 5 MINUTES

No cooking or blending is required to make this easy salad dressing. Just shake and enjoy! We use this in our Pomegranate, Poppy Seed, and Spinach Salad (page 102).

3 tablespoons extra-virgin olive oil

2 tablespoons white vinegar

2 tablespoons white sugar

1 teaspoon poppy seeds

¼ teaspoon salt

¼ teaspoon smooth Dijon mustard or

   ⅛ teaspoon ground mustard

In a salad dressing shaker, combine the oil, vinegar, sugar, poppy seeds, salt, and mustard. Shake well to emulsify. Store the leftovers in the refrigerator for up to 2 weeks. Shake before using.

VARIATION TIP: Canola oil or another mild-tasting oil can be used instead of olive oil. Apple cider vinegar or freshly squeezed lemon juice can be used instead of white vinegar.

INGREDIENT TIP: When stored in the refrigerator, olive oil can turn solid. It will return to liquid when it is at room temperature again.

Per Serving (1 tablespoon):
Calories: 119; Total Fat: 11g; Saturated Fat: 2g; Cholesterol: 0mg; Sodium: 151mg; Carbohydrates: 6g; Fiber: 0g; Protein: 0g

References

Barrett, Jacqueline S. "How to Institute the Low-FODMAP Diet." *Journal of Gastroenterology and Hepatology* 32, S1 (February 2017): 8–10. https://doi.org/10.1111/jgh.13686.

Canadian Digestive Health Foundation. "Signs and Symptoms." Accessed August 16, 2019. https://cdhf.ca/digestive-disorders/irritable-bowel-syndrome-ibs/signs-and -symptoms/.

Celiac Disease Foundation. "Testing & Diagnosis." Accessed August 15, 2019. https://celiac.org/about-celiac-disease/screening-and-diagnosis/.

De Bortoli, Nicola, Irene Martinucci, Massimo Bellini, Edoardo Savarino, Vincenzo Savarino, Corrado Blandizi, and Santino Marchi. "Overlap of Functional Heartburn and Gastroesophageal Reflux Disease with Irritable Bowel Syndrome." *World Journal of Gastroenterology* 19, 35 (September 2013): 5787–97. https://www.ncbi.nlm.nih.gov/ pmc/articles/PMC3793133/.

Dietitians of Canada. "Learn about Dietitians." Accessed August 16, 2019. https://www .dietitians.ca/About-Us/About-Dietitians/Learn-about-Dietitians.aspx.

El-Salhy, Magdy, Synne Otterasen Ystad, Tarek Mazzawi, and Doris Gundersen. "Dietary Fiber in Irritable Bowel Syndrome (Review)." *International Journal of Molecular Medicine* 40, 3 (September 2017): 607–13. https://doi.org/10.3892/ijmm.2017.3072.

Everyday Nutrition. "Does Your Period Make IBS Worse?" November 2, 2018. Accessed August 16, 2019. https://everydaynutrition.com.au/does-your-period-make-ibs-worse/.

FODMAP Friendly. "FODMAP Friendly." Google Play, Vers 9.5 (2019). Accessed August 16, 2019. https://play.google.com/store/apps/details?id=com.foodmap.

Foster, Jane A., Linda Rinaman, and John F. Cryan. "Stress & the Gut-Brain Axis: Regulation by the Microbiome." *Neurobiology of Stress* 7 (December 2017): 124–36. https://doi.org/10.1016/j.ynstr.2017.03.001.

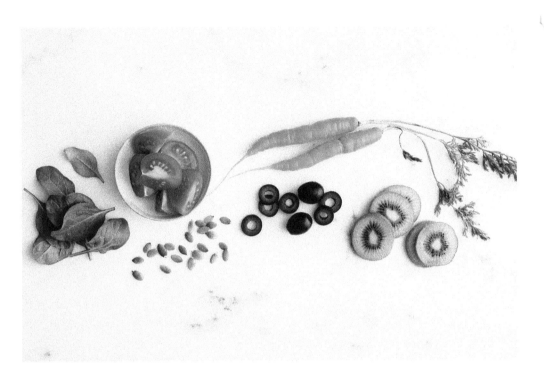

Furnari, Manuele, Nicola de Bortoli, Irene Martinucci, Giorgia Bodini, Matteo Revelli, Elisa Marabotto, Alessandro Moscatelli, Lorenzo Del Nero, et al. "Optimal Management of Constipation Associated with Irritable Bowel Syndrome." *Therapeutics and Clinical Risk Management 11* (2015): 691–703. https://doi.org/10.2147/TCRM.S54298.

Gastrointestinal Society. "Constipation Overview." Accessed August 16, 2019. https://badgut.org/information-centre/a-z-digestive-topics/constipation/.

Gibson, Peter R. "The Evidence Base for Efficacy of the Low FODMAP Diet in Irritable Bowel Syndrome: Is It Ready for Prime Time as a First-Line Therapy?" *Journal of Gastroenterology and Hepatology* 32, S1 (February 2017): 32–35. https://doi.org/10.1111/jgh.13693.

Iacovou, Marina. "Adapting the Low FODMAP Diet to Special Populations: Infants and Children." *Journal of Gastroenterology and Hepatology* 32, S1 (February 2017): 43–45. https://doi.org/10.1111/jgh.13696.

Ignite Nutrition. "Nutrition & SIBO." February 28, 2019. Accessed August 16, 2019. https://ignitenutrition.ca/blog/nutrition-sibo/.

Inouye, Audrey. "Dining Out on the Low FODMAP Diet." *IBS Nutrition.* December 19, 2018. Accessed August 15, 2019. http://www.ibsnutrition.com/dining-low-fodmap-diet/.

Lacy, Brian E., and Nihal K. Patel. "Rome Criteria and a Diagnostic Approach to Irritable Bowel Syndrome." *Journal of Clinical Medicine* 6, 11 (2017): 99. https://doi.org/10.3390/jcm6110099.

Lucak, Susan, Lin Chang, Albena Halpert, and Lucinda A. Harris. "Current and Emergent Pharmacologic Treatments for Irritable Bowel Syndrome with Diarrhea: Evidence-Based Treatment in Practice." *Therapeutic Advances in Gastroenterology* 10, 2 (2016): 253–75. https://doi.org/10.1177/1756283X16663396.

Monash University. "Update: Bananas Re-tested!" Accessed August 16, 2019. https://www.monashfodmap.com/blog/update-bananas-re-tested/.

Monash University. "Endometriosis and IBS—Why the Low FODMAP Diet May Become Part of the Treatment." Accessed August 16, 2019. https://www.monashfodmap.com/blog/endometriosis-and-ibs-why-low-fodmap/.

Monash University. "High and Low FODMAP Foods." Accessed August 15, 2019. https://www.monashfodmap.com/about-fodmap-and-ibs/high-and-low-fodmap-foods/.

Monash University. "Let's Talk Number Twos—What's 'Normal' and When Should I Worry?" Accessed August 15, 2019. https://www.monashfodmap.com/blog/lets-talk-number-twos-whats-normal-and/.

Monash University. "Monash University Low FODMAP Diet." Google Play, Vers.3.0.3 (2019). Accessed on August 16, 2019. https://play.google.com/store/apps/details?id=com.monashuniversity.fodmap&hl=en.

Monash University. "The 3 Steps of the FODMAP Diet." Accessed August 15, 2019. https://www.monashfodmap.com/blog/3-phases-low-fodmap-diet/.

National Institute for Health and Care Excellence. "Irritable Bowel Syndrome in Adults: Diagnosis and Management: Guidance." Last modified April 2017. https://www.nice.org.uk/guidance/cg61.

Niv, E., A. Halak, E. Tiommny, H. Yanai, H. Strul, T. Naftali, and N. Vaisman. "Randomized Clinical Study: Partially Hydrolyzed Guar Gum (PHGG) versus Placebo in the Treatment of Patients with Irritable Bowel Syndrome." *Nutrition & Metabolism* 13, 10 (June 2016). https://doi.org/10.1186/s12986-016-0070-5.

O'Keeffe, Majella, and Miranda CE Lomer. "Who Should Deliver the Low FODMAP Diet and What Educational Methods Are Optimal: A Review." *Journal of Gastroenterology and Hepatology* 32, S1 (2017): 23–26. https://doi.org/10.1111/jgh.13690.

Peters, S. L., C. K. Yao, H. Philpott, G. W. Yelland, J. G. Muir, and P. R. Gibson. "Randomised Clinical Trial: The Efficacy of Gut-Directed Hypnotherapy Is Similar to That of the Low FODMAP Diet for the Treatment of Irritable Bowel Syndrome." *Alimentary Pharmacology & Therapeutics* 44, 5 (2016): 447–59. https://doi.org/10.1111/apt.13706.

Renlund, Lauren. "FODMAP Content of Tea (and Easy Recipe for Fresh Ginger Maple Tea)." Last modified January 26, 2017. http://www.laurenrenlund.com/2017/01/26/fodmap-content-of-tea-easy-fresh-ginger-maple-tea-recipe/.

Roncoroni, Leda, Karla A. Bascuñán, Luisa Doneda, Alice Scricciolo, Vincenza Lombardo, Federica Branchi, Francesca Ferretti, et al. "Correction: Roncoroni, L. et al. A Low FODMAP Gluten-Free Diet Improves Functional Gastrointestinal Disorders and Overall Mental Health of Celiac Disease Patients: A Randomized Controlled Trial. *Nutrients* 2018, 10, 1023." *Nutrients* 11, 3 (2019): 566. https://doi.org/10.3390/nu11030566.

Schwille-Kiuntke, J., N. Mazurak, and P. Enck. "Systematic Review with Meta-Analysis: Post-Infectious Irritable Bowel Syndrome after Travellers' Diarrhoea." *Alimentary Pharmacology & Therapeutics* 41, 11 (April 2015): 1029–37. https://doi.org/10.1111/apt.13199.

Spiller, Robin. "How Do FODMAPs Work?" *Journal of Gastroenterology and Hepatology* 32, S1 (February 2017): 36–39. https://doi.org/10.1111/jgh.13694.

The American Academy of Allergy, Asthma & Immunology. "The Myth of IgG Food Panel Testing." Accessed August 15, 2019. https://www.aaaai.org/conditions-and-treatments/library/allergy-library/IgG-food-test.

Tuck, Caroline, and Jacqueline Barrett. "Re-Challenging FODMAPs: The Low FODMAP Diet Phase Two." *Journal of Gastroenterology and Hepatology* 32, S1 (February 2017): 11–15. https://doi.org/10.1111/jgh.13687.

Tuck, Caroline J., Kirstin M. Taylor, Jacqueline Barrett, Peter R. Gibson, and Jane Muir. "Oral Galactosidase Improves Gastrointestinal Tolerance to a Diet High in Galacto-Oligosaccharides: Adjunct Therapy to a Low FODMAP Diet in Irritable Bowel Syndrome." *Gastroenterology* 152, 5 (April 2017): S45. https://doi.org/10.1016/s0016-5085(17)30514-0.

United States Department of Agriculture Food Safety and Inspection Service. "Keep Food Safe! Food Safety Basics." Accessed August 15, 2019. https://bit.ly/2GE10Fh.

Varney, Jane, Jacqueline Barrett, Kate Scarlata, Patsy Catsos, Peter R. Gibson, and Jane G. Muir. "FODMAPs: Food Composition, Defining Cutoff Values and International Application." *Journal of Gastroenterology and Hepatology* 32, S1 (February 2017): 53–61. https://doi.org/10.1111/jgh.13698.

Wang, Ben, Ruqiao Duan, and Liping Duan. "Prevalence of Sleep Disorder in Irritable Bowel Syndrome: A Systematic Review with Meta-Analysis." *The Saudi Journal of Gastroenterology* 24, 3 (2018): 141–50. https://doi.org/10.4103/sjg.sjg_603_17.

Low-FODMAP Resources

WEBSITES

A Little Bit Yummy (www.ALittleBitYummy.com): A Little Bit Yummy was founded by Alana Scott after she was diagnosed with celiac disease and irritable bowel syndrome. Alana's mission is to help you fall back in love with food again with low-FODMAP recipes and resources that are dietitian-reviewed so you can eat with confidence. This website is a go-to resource if you need meal plans, up-to-date information on the low-FODMAP diet, recipe inspiration, and support.

Everyday Nutrition (www.EverydayNutrition.com.au): Joanna Baker is a Monash FODMAP–trained Australia-based accredited practicing dietitian, registered nurse, and foodie who is passionate about digestive health. She works exclusively with people with IBS and food intolerance in her Melbourne-based private practice, Everyday Nutrition.

FODY Foods (www.FodyFoods.com): Fody Foods is the first company to offer an entire range of Monash-certified, low-FODMAP, gluten-free, and vegan products for all eating occasions ranging from snacks to sauces, condiments, and more. They are committed to bringing back the joy in eating for those suffering with IBS and other digestive disorders.

The Global Dietitian (www.TheGlobalDietitian.com): Diana Reid is a Monash FODMAP-trained, Europe-based registered dietitian who specializes in gut health, pediatric and adolescent nutrition, sports nutrition, and general wellness.

IBS Nutrition (www.IBSNutrition.com): Audrey Inouye, RD, is a Monash FODMAP–trained Canada-based registered dietitian who specializes in IBS. Her nutrition practice is in Edmonton, Alberta, where she provides in-person support and virtual services across Canada. You can also find IBS nutrition on Facebook and Instagram @IBSNutrition.

International Foundation for Functional Gastrointestinal Disorders (IFFGD) (www.IFFGD.org): The mission of the IFFGD is to inform, assist, and support people affected by gastrointestinal disorders.

Kate Watson, RD (www.KateWatsonRD.com): Kate Watson is a Monash FODMAP-trained, US-based registered dietitian. She specializes in IBS and SIBO and offers virtual services throughout the United States and in person in Edmonds, Washington, USA.

Lauren Renlund, MPH, RD (www.LaurenRenlund.com): Lauren was diagnosed with IBS in 2014 and uses a modified low-FODMAP diet to manage her symptoms. She is a FODMAP specialist dietitian and loves helping others with IBS by sharing delicious recipes and helpful tips online.

Monash University (www.MonashFODMAP.com): The low-FODMAP diet was specially developed by Monash University researchers to provide relief from IBS. The Monash FODMAP website contains links to their app, blog, recipe directory, dietitian directory, and online training for dietitians.

BOOK

Bloated Belly Whisperer, **Tamara Duker Freuman, MS, RD, CDN** (www.TheBloatedBellyWhisperer.com): An evidence-based self-help guide for people who experience bloating of an unknown cause. The book covers the 10 most common causes of abdominal bloating and distension and is written by a registered dietitian from a leading New York gastroenterology practice.

Index

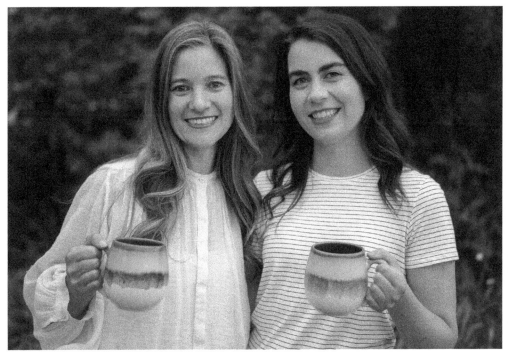

Photo by Garrett Rokosh

Our Acknowledgments

We would like to thank our network of FODMAP specialist dietitians from around the world for their support, with a special acknowledgment to Joanna Baker, APD, and Kate Watson, RD. In addition, Alana Scott from A Little Bit Yummy is always immensely helpful and was always available when we needed to reach out.

Thank you to all our patients, who have taught us so much. Thank you to anyone who has ever read our blogs or participated in our Low FODMAP Canadians Facebook group.

AUDREY'S ACKNOWLEDGMENTS

A special thank you to my husband, Dave, for being my biggest fan and always encouraging me to do what makes me happy. You have convinced me to do things that I never dreamed of, like travel around the world with our young kids (twice), learn how to surf, and write a cookbook.

To my three boys, my most critical recipe testers: Thank you for having really big appetites and rating all of my recipes with wholehearted honesty.

To my dear friend Lauren, I have loved working side by side with you on yet another project. I will forever be impressed with you and your accomplishments in life.

LAUREN'S ACKNOWLEDGMENTS

Thank you to my friends and my whole family. Your endless support means the world to me.

Eric, you are a wonderful brother, and I am so grateful to have you in my life. Mom and Dad, I have a fulfilling career and life today because of you; your unconditional love and support have allowed me to chase my dreams and live my best life. Grandma, you inspire me every day to think creatively and live healthfully. Grandpa and Nana, although you are gone, your love for food continues to inspire me.

Audrey, thank you for being like a big sister to me. I have loved working with you from the start of my career and am excited for all the things yet to come!

About the Authors

Audrey Inouye, BSc, RD, Monash FODMAP–Trained Dietitian

Audrey is a Canada-based Monash FODMAP-trained dietitian, owner of www.IBSNutrition.com, a soccer mom, and a travel addict. Her practice is in Edmonton, Alberta, where she provides in-person support and virtual services across Canada. You can find Audrey on Facebook and Instagram @IBSNutrition. Audrey is married, with three boys and a new puppy.

Lauren Renlund, BASc, MPH, RD

Lauren is a Canadian dietitian and food lover. She was diagnosed with IBS in 2014 and uses a modified low-FODMAP diet to manage her symptoms. She recently moved to Edmonton, Alberta, where she loves spending her free time drinking tea, exploring the outdoors, laughing with friends, and daydreaming about food.

Printed in the USA
CPSIA information can be obtained
at www.ICGtesting.com
LVHW052135091223
765798LV00002B/16